Drug Testing
in Correctional Settings

Drug Testing in Correctional Settings

GUIDELINES FOR EFFECTIVE USE

■ ■ ■

Robert L. DuPont, M.D.

Thomas M. Mieczkowski, Ph.D.

Richard A. Newel, Ph.D.

HAZELDEN®

Hazelden
Center City, Minnesota 55012-0176

1-800-328-9000
1-651-213-4590 (Fax)
www.hazelden.org

To request permission, write to Permissions Coordinator, Hazelden, P.O. Box 176, Center City, MN 55012-0176. To purchase additional copies of this publication, call 1-800-328-9000 or 1-651-213-4000.

ISBN-13: 978-1-59285-181-2
ISBN-10: 1-59285-181-9

09 08 07 06 05   6 5 4 3 2 1

Editor's note: While the authors have made every effort to be accurate based on the latest information available, facts and legal issues change and may need the review of attorneys and suppliers of drug tests.

Cover design by Theresa Gedig
Interior design and typesetting by Kinne Design

Contents

■   ■   ■

Acknowledgments

■   ■   ■

We wish to thank our families and our colleagues for the help that they have provided us in writing this manual. We thank the countless professionals with whom we have worked over the past decades in the criminal justice system and in drug-abuse treatment. In particular, we thank the offenders with whom we have worked who have used drug testing as a major support for their recovery from addiction. Their experiences have been our inspiration. Thanks to the John P. McGovern Foundation for support of this project through the Institute for Behavior and Health, Inc.

In writing this manual, we have had valuable assistance from Audrey Bumanis, who managed the writing process from start to finish as three authors and several editors worked on this manuscript. She has pulled off this near miracle with skill and a sense of humor that has made the long hours of writing seem both less long and more fun. We would also like to thank Paul Brethen, M.A., M.F.T., for his contributions regarding evaluation and research in Hazelden's *Drug Testing in Treatment Settings*. We used that text as a guide in developing a similar chapter in this manual.

We thank Hazelden for asking us to write this manual. Hazelden is distinguished in the history of our country's response to the serious problem of addiction in two remarkable ways. First, Hazelden set the standard for modern addiction treatment by pioneering the revolutionary Minnesota Model of drug-abuse treatment. To promote lifelong recovery, this influential model of addiction treatment features individualized treatment plans using residential and outpatient services from dedicated professional therapists, some of whom are themselves in recovery, as well as intensive and prolonged involvement with Twelve Step programs.

Second, for half a century Hazelden has been the nation's leading publisher of materials related to addiction and recovery. It is an honor for us to have this manual published by Hazelden. The staff at Hazelden with whom we have worked closely on this manual has provided valuable guidance and skilled editorial assistance at every step of the process from our first outline to the last correction of our faulty sentences. We thank in particular Sue Thomas, Karen Chernyaev, Corrine Casanova, and Tracy Lutz.

The errors that no doubt remain in this manual are our responsibility. We have endeavored to make this manual accurate, reader-friendly, and useful. As practitioners who ourselves have worked with great satisfaction for many years in the criminal justice system, we are aware of just how big, complex, and important this too-often-maligned nonsystem system really is. We are deeply grateful to the many people who have dedicated their professional lives to helping criminal offenders become productive, law-abiding, and reasonably happy members of our communities. These criminal justice professionals are the unsung heroes of America's crime-prevention efforts. It is to them that we dedicate this manual.

■   ■   ■

1

■　■　■　■　■

Introduction

The drug-abuse epidemic began in the United States in the late 1960s with a shock wave of heroin addiction that dramatically drove up the rate of serious crimes and flooded our nation's prisons. Later, in the mid-1980s, the crack cocaine epidemic hit the nation with devastating force. This one-two battering had overwhelming effects on the criminal justice system. As the nation came face-to-face with the epidemic of illegal drug use in the 1990s, there was a bipartisan effort to toughen sentences and to reduce judicial discretion in sentencing for drug offenses and other crimes. Today, the nation's criminal justice system is awash in illegal drugs as the prison population has reached alarming levels resulting in high costs as well as painful political dilemmas.

Intense controversies about national drug policy have zeroed in on the role of the criminal justice system. Some critics have stridently posed the policy choice facing the nation today as "treatment versus prison" for illegal drug users. After long careers in drug-abuse treatment and the criminal justice system, we see the most important choice about drugs facing our country quite differently. To us, the most important drug-abuse policy question that needs to be answered in dealing with crime and drug use in the criminal justice system is not whether to choose treatment or prison. Rather, it is this: how can the criminal justice system and the new national drug-abuse treatment system better work together to curb illegal drug use and to reduce crime? More than

60 percent of the drug abusers now in treatment in this country are there because of the criminal justice system. This statistic alone gives new meaning to the claim that the only policy choice is treatment or prison. Without the authority of the criminal justice system, drug-treatment programs in this country would shrink by more than half.

> For millions of American drug abusers who wind up in the criminal justice system, it is their last, best hope of not only getting well but of staying well from the progressive and potentially fatal disease of addiction.

For millions of American drug abusers who wind up in the criminal justice system, it is their last, best hope of not only getting well but of staying well from the progressive and potentially fatal disease of addiction. For that goal to be achieved, however, it is vitally important that the criminal justice system enforce a drug-free standard throughout the offenders' periods of supervision from pretrial release to probation, prison, and parole. Once that standard of abstinence is set and enforced, the lifesaving and ultimately joyful process of recovery can begin. That is where treatment comes into the picture. Drug-abuse treatment is one good way for offenders to meet the requirement of the criminal justice system that they stay drug free. Abstinence-based Twelve Step programs such as Alcoholics Anonymous (AA) and Narcotics Anonymous (NA), while not "treatment," can also play important roles in sustaining robust recovery.

In the last decade, the establishment of drug courts has not only captured the nation's attention, but also has brought together the key elements that are necessary for the criminal justice system to fulfill its potential as a major agent of drug-abuse prevention and treatment. These elements include abstinence enforced by drug tests while upholding the shared goal of a crime-free and drug-free life. To achieve this goal, drug courts typically make extensive use of both treatment and frequent attendance at Twelve Step meetings, along with relatively prolonged and intensive periods of supervision.

This manual is written for everyone in the criminal justice system who wants to help criminal offenders stay off drugs in order to give them a better chance to live crime-free lives. Drug testing is a significant tool in achieving this goal. However, to achieve the full potential of modern drug testing, the criminal justice system has to get smarter than it is today. Drug testing is not only the pinnacle of modern biotechnology, it is also evolving rapidly to become cheaper, easier to use, and able to test a wider range of abused substances. To achieve the potential of today's drug-testing technologies, the criminal justice system needs to get beyond the urine cup and use the full range of on-site and laboratory-based drug tests with flexibility and sophistication.

Doing this will help the criminal justice system achieve its twin goals of preventing illegal drug use and intervening strongly with drug treatment. Drug testing is a powerful prevention tool precisely because it breaks through denial and dishonesty. When criminal offenders are drug tested wisely and often, they know that sustained return to drug use will be detected. They know that the consequences of positive drug tests will be imposed on them and that these consequences will be swift, serious, and certain.

The secondary but still important goal of drug testing in the criminal justice system is to identify early sustained return to illegal drug use so that effective interventions can be made to stop the drug use quickly. This is a matter not only of protecting the community from drug-caused crime but also a matter of life and death for illegal drug users. If community corrections, including halfway houses, parole, and probation, is to deserve the support of the crime-fearing public, then agencies of the criminal justice system must be able to ensure that those offenders under their supervision are drug free. Drug testing can play a key role in establishing this assurance.

> The secondary but still important goal of drug testing in the criminal justice system is to identify early sustained return to illegal drug use so that effective interventions can be made to stop the drug use quickly.

This manual is written to provide an overview of all the key information that is needed to successfully implement a drug-testing program in a correctional setting. Chapter 2 of this manual gives an overview of the history behind drug testing and explains why drug testing is needed in the criminal justice system. It provides a context in which to understand the role of drug testing. Chapter 3 explains how drug testing can be used in the many settings of the criminal justice system. It provides practical help to program managers and to the people who are using drug testing to maximize the potential of this remarkable biotechnology. Chapter 4 gives an overview of the science behind drug testing and the pros and cons of each type of drug test. We will explore the opportunities to use a variety of new drug-testing strategies, including testing for abused drugs in hair, oral fluids, and sweat. Because drug testing is rapidly evolving, we focus on state-of-the-art science and practice and look to the future of drug testing as well.

Building on this solid foundation, we then turn in chapter 5 to a range of practical issues such as determining the most efficient ways to manage a drug-testing program, starting with how to test, when to test, how often to test, and how to handle positive drug-test results. Here you will also find practical suggestions for improving the effectiveness and lowering the costs of drug testing.

In chapter 6, we look at ways to solve many of the common problems that are associated with drug testing, including cheating, dealing with the poppy-seed problem, and managing and evaluating claims that a positive drug test was wrong.

Finally, in chapter 7, we explore evaluation, research, and program improvements to be made over time in operating drug-testing programs and conclude with a review of additional sources of useful information and support.

This manual is both a resource to help solve the problems that emerge in the interpretation of drug-test results and a guide to the development and improvement of drug-testing programs in the criminal justice system. In particular, we aim to meet the needs of law-enforcement officers and jail, prison, probation, and parole staff, as well as the courts and judges who are the most frequent consumers of drug-test results.

> This manual is both a resource to help solve the problems that emerge in the interpretation of drug-test results and a guide to the development and improvement of drug-testing programs in the criminal justice system.

2

■ ■ ■ ■ ■

The History of and Need for Drug Testing in Correctional Settings

A Brief History of Drug Testing

Drug testing began more than fifty years ago as part of death investigations in medical examiners' offices. It was a time-consuming, expensive process that was seldom used. In the 1960s, drug testing began to be used in the then-new civil commitment drug-abuse treatment programs in California and New York. Drug testing for heroin was used to keep tabs on offenders' drug use, both as a way to measure their progress in recovery as well as a way to watch for relapse. Only in the 1970s did drug testing become widespread in the criminal justice system and drug-abuse treatment programs, especially in the methadone treatment programs that were then becoming common in all parts of the country.

The most important new use of drug testing came in June of 1971 when the U.S. military began testing soldiers returning from overseas, especially Vietnam, for heroin addiction. It had been discovered that illegal drug use was a serious threat to the readiness of U.S. forces. Military personnel who tested positive for recent heroin use were sent to drug-treatment programs where they were constantly drug tested to evaluate their progress and motivate them to stay clean. A clean urine test was required before being allowed to return home.

In the early 1980s, public outcry over the problems related to drug abuse, particularly after the crash on the aircraft carrier USS *Nimitz* in 1981 and the subsequent high levels of drug use found among navy personnel, led to a growing interest in extending drug testing to nonclinical populations. The dramatic effect of instituting a drug-testing program among all military personnel was seen when soldiers reported that their drug use in the past thirty days fell from 28 percent in 1980 to 5 percent in 1988. As a result, when the devastating crack cocaine epidemic began in 1986, one of the responses nationwide was to institute the use of drug testing in the civilian workplace. Today, drug testing in the civilian workforce is primarily limited to pre-employment testing and testing in safety- and security-sensitive jobs, especially those related to the nuclear power industry and among commercial drivers. Some private employers use random drug testing for all employees as well.

> Today, drug testing in the civilian workforce is primarily limited to pre-employment testing and testing in safety- and security-sensitive jobs.

Following a landmark Supreme Court decision in 1995, drug testing has become increasingly common in the nation's schools. Student drug testing, like testing in the military and in the civilian workplace, is part of a comprehensive drug-abuse prevention strategy.

Drug testing is also used in many health care settings, including emergency-room evaluations. In many public mental health centers, drug testing is also routine because of the high rates of comorbidity of major mental illness and substance-use disorders.

Wherever drug abuse is a significant problem, drug testing is now used. Drug testing is highly effective in identifying recent drug use, which is essential to helping drug users get the help that they need to overcome their drug problems. If continuing illegal drug use is not identified, the purposes of helping institutions—including those in the criminal justice system—are endangered. The only objective way to identify recent illegal drug use is with drug tests. If drug testing is not done frequently and systematically, then most ongoing illegal drug use will not be identified in whatever population is being served.

> Wherever drug abuse is a significant problem, drug testing is now used.

The future of drug testing is easy to predict: there will be more of it in more settings. Drug testing will expand to include on-site breath tests for a wide range of drugs of abuse. Drug tests in the future will continue to get better and cheaper as they are more widely used. More organizations doing drug testing will extend their testing beyond traditional urine testing to take advantage of the newer alternative testing opportunities, including the testing of hair, oral fluids, and sweat.

Establishing the Need for Drug Testing in Correctional Settings

Drug testing and the criminal justice system have a history dating back about three decades. The first citywide criminal justice system drug-testing program involved not only pretrial but also parole and probation. Begun in the nation's capital, it is run by the Superior Court. That historic drug-testing program, called the District of Columbia Pretrial Services Agency, has been in continuous operation since 1970 and is directed by Susan W. Shaffer, Esq.

> Drug testing and the criminal justice system have a history dating back about three decades.

The interest in drug testing in correctional settings was fueled by the same general concern about the rapid and dramatic rise in drug use that caused other social institutions, like the workplace and the military, to institute drug testing. The alarm over the rapidly rising rates of illegal drug use and crime was linked to another important development, this one technical. The establishment of immunoassay technology—the use of the antibody/antigen reaction in clinical chemistry—made possible rapid and relatively low-cost drug testing for the first time. Linking these two developments together largely accounts for the initiation and establishment of drug testing within the criminal justice system.

As drug-abuse treatment and criminal justice evolved over the past decades, so did drug tests. Early drug tests could identify only a few drugs and only when the drugs were present at very high concentrations. They all used urine. From that foundation, drug tests have evolved to the point today where virtually all drugs of abuse can be identified by drug tests, and the drugs can be identified at very low concentrations. Recent drug use can now be identified not just in urine, but in many body fluids, including blood, sweat, and saliva (oral fluids) as well as in hair, fingernails, and virtually all other parts of the body of the drug user. Breath testing is also common for alcohol.

Why Is the Criminal Justice System Involved in Drug Testing?

Drug abuse can be seen from many perspectives—for example, as a public health problem, a crime problem, or a moral issue. Why is the criminal justice system so swept up in the phenomenon of drug abuse and the societal response to drug abuse?

People working in the criminal justice system might consider it odd to ask the question. We have come to naturally link crime, criminal law enforcement, arrest, and incarceration with drug distribution, use, and abuse. Why is this so? Start by considering that the number of persons arrested for drug offenses has tripled over the last two decades (see figure 1), outstripping every other form of criminal offense category.

> The number of persons arrested for drug offenses has tripled over the last two decades, outstripping every other form of criminal offense category.

FIGURE 1

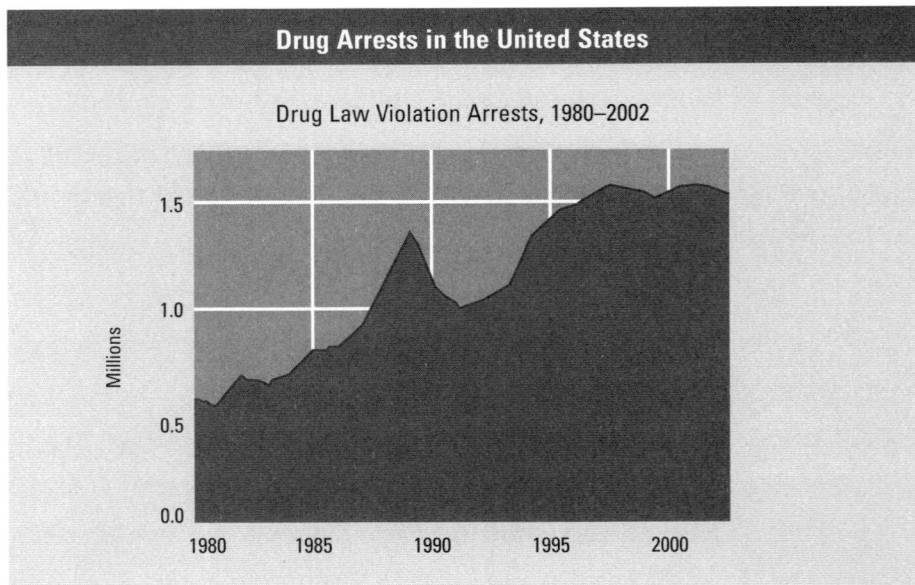

Drug Arrests in the United States

Drug Law Violation Arrests, 1980–2002

From the Federal Bureau of Investigation, Uniform Crime Reports, www.fbi.gov/ucr/ucr.htm, 2002

During that time span, arrests for drug offenses have increased at a phenomenal rate and so have the subsequent charges, the criminal processing, and ultimately the convictions and sentencing associated with these arrests. The number of persons incarcerated in prison for drug offenses increased an astounding 1,195 percent from 1980 to 2001 (19,000 in 1980 to 246,100 in 2001). The number of drug offenders was about the same as public order offenders in the early 1980s. From 1984 to 1990, the number of drug offenders rose dramatically, increasing by more than 50 percent from 1988 to 1989 alone. By 1990, the number of drug offenders was similar to the number of property offenders (Bureau of Justice Statistics, *Correctional Populations in the United States, Annual* and *Prisoners in 2002*).

> The number of persons incarcerated in prison for drug offenses increased an astounding 1,195 percent from 1980 to 2001.

Not only are the numbers of incarcerated drug offenders rising, but according to the Bureau of Justice Statistics, about 25 percent of all probationers in state correctional custody are under supervision for drug-law violations. This comes to nearly 500,000 persons in the United States who are in prison or on parole or probation for drug offenses. When excluding violent offenses in the correctional population, drug offenses dwarf all other categories of offenses. Drug offenses even outperformed *all* other nonviolent property offenses *combined* in the year 2000. Figure 2 illustrates the dominant role that drug offenses have come to occupy within our justice system.

FIGURE 2

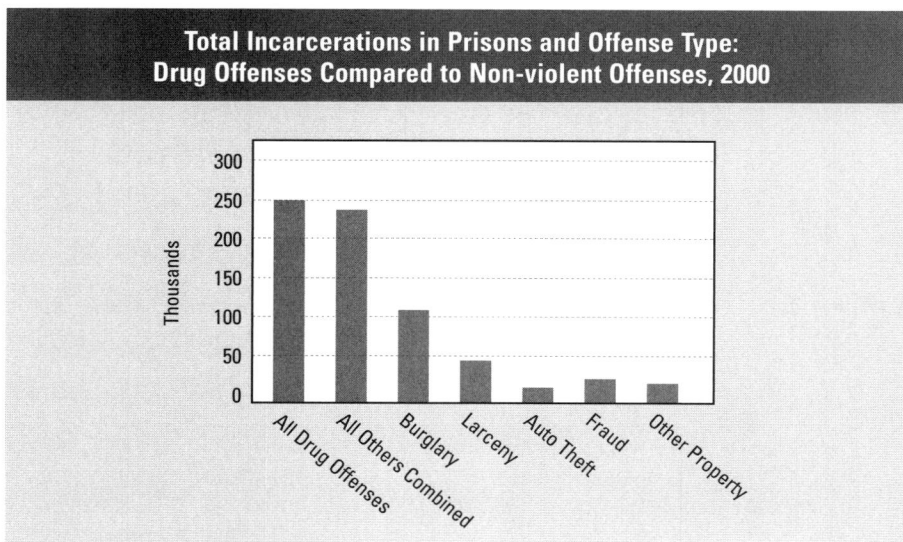

Total Incarcerations in Prisons and Offense Type: Drug Offenses Compared to Non-violent Offenses, 2000

From the Bureau of Justice Statistics, 2000

Effectively dealing with the drug problem in the criminal justice system achieves four important objectives. First, it significantly reduces crime since drug abuse is one of the prime drivers of criminal behavior. Second, it reduces the level of drug abuse in the community at large because a significant number of the heaviest drug users are caught up in the criminal justice system. Third, it reduces the drug market by removing many of the biggest consumers of drugs. Fourth, and perhaps most important to us, the leverage of the criminal justice system, when applied to individual drug abusers, can literally save their lives from the ravages of drug abuse by effectively promoting long-lasting recovery.

Due to this large presence of drug abusers in the criminal justice system, the need for drug testing is great. Drug testing is an effective tool in supporting the treatment and long-term recovery of drug-abusing offenders.

> Effectively dealing with the drug problem in the criminal justice system achieves four important objectives.

3

. . . . .

How Drug Testing Can Be Used
in Correctional Settings

One of the hallmarks of addiction is denial. Drug testing is the ultimate denial buster. Some critics see drug testing as unduly intrusive. On the contrary, to permit an offender to stay in the community without ongoing random drug testing is not only harmful to the offender, but to the community as a whole. Drug testing is compassionate because it helps offenders become and remain drug free. It promotes honesty and accountability while effectively defusing the often emotionally charged assessment and supervision process. Drug testing is a valuable tool throughout the full spectrum of supervision in the criminal justice system.

Drug testing largely targets two groups in the criminal justice system. One group is persons who come in contact with the system as a consequence of a legal confrontation with authorities resulting in arrest. In these cases, drug testing is done at intake so that drug courts and pretrial release programs can establish whether the offender has recently used specific drugs of abuse. Continuous drug testing is then done to help determine the subsequent levels of drugs used by each offender and to help the courts determine what, if any, sanctions (including incarceration) may be needed as part of that person's recovery.

Another target group is persons who are in custody as probationers, parolees, or convicts. Offenders who are released into the community under state supervision are subject to drug testing "on demand." This type of drug testing acts as a powerful deterrent to continued drug use. Positive drug-test results discovered by a probation or parole officer can lead to a violation and incarceration. In these circumstances drug abstinence becomes an enforceable requirement. The community and the judiciary are more likely to support release back into the community if the community can be assured that violations of release conditions can be accurately detected and punished. Regular, systematic drug testing helps to provide that assurance, which is a necessary condition of all community-based criminal justice programs.

> Another target group is persons who are in custody as probationers, parolees, or convicts.

The Legality of Drug Testing in Correctional Settings

Prior to being found guilty, persons under arrest generally cannot be forced into a drug test unless a court warrant is obtained. This has been established by the courts for any "invasive" testing. Invasive testing has typically referred to the examination of anything retained in the body, such as urine or blood. Whether this would apply to hair or saliva is not clear. More often than not, persons who have been arrested but not yet convicted or even charged with a crime cannot be forced to undergo testing without a court warrant. A drug test is considered a legal "search," and the protection of citizens from illegal search and seizure usually applies. Persons convicted of a crime, however, have more limited rights and generally can be tested at the will of their jailers/wardens. Persons who consent voluntarily can always be tested.

A conservative interpretation would be that persons who are arrested probably cannot be forced to undergo a drug test without a court order, although they may consent to one if they are offered inducements to undergo testing (i.e., if it makes them eligible for early release or bonding). Once a person is convicted, they are subject to testing without much, if any, limitation.

> It is desirable for any program doing drug testing in the criminal justice system to have the program's attorneys review the legal status of drug testing since there are many state, local, and federal laws involved and because the law is constantly changing.

It is desirable for any program doing drug testing in the criminal justice system to have the program's attorneys review the legal status of drug testing since there are many state, local, and federal laws involved and because the law is constantly changing.

Following is a more detailed description of how drug testing can be used in a variety of correctional settings.

Drug Testing to Help with Planning

How Many People Are Using What Types of Drugs?

When criminal justice jurisdictions plan for the number of people who will need special services for addiction, they often conduct surveys to find out the answers to two questions: How many of our offenders use drugs? And what types of drugs are they using? Criminal justice agencies often begin these drug epidemiology studies by examining existing records of the number of drug arrests and convictions, sometimes sampling arrest records to get an idea of the proportion of offenders using specific drugs.

Answering these questions can be more difficult than it would first appear because many illegal drug users requiring special services do not have a primary charge of drug possession or sales. Often they are charged for property crimes such as burglary or violent crimes such as murder. Criminal justice professionals know that both of these crimes are often the result of involvement with drugs.

Also, simply watching drug arrests, for example cocaine arrests, over time can be deceptive since it may be confounded by special tactics and enforcement programs that target an area known to be a high drug-use area over a limited amount of time. This would give the impression that drug use is skyrocketing, even though the sudden rise in the number of arrests is directly due to a concentrated effort in law enforcement.

More productive than simply reviewing arrest records are the studies (using drug testing) conducted at intake facilities at local jails. This research began as the National Institute of Justice's Drug Use Forecasting (DUF) study and ran for many years in dozens of cities nationwide. Known more recently as the Arrestee Drug Abuse Monitoring (ADAM) program, it was discontinued due to lack of funding in 2004. However, the strategy of collecting voluntary drug use reports and urine samples from arrestees as they are being booked

> More productive than simply reviewing arrest records are the studies (using drug testing) conducted at intake facilities at local jails.

into a local jail has been emulated by sheriff's departments and city jails nationwide. Over time, the information obtained from these self-reports and drug tests depicts the rate of positive drug samples for each drug of concern among the offenders who volunteer to be tested as part of their booking procedures.

Although volunteers are used, most of the people approached in a jail setting are willing to give a urine sample provided they are assured that the results of the drug test are for research and evaluation only and will not be used against them. Often their only reward for participation is a break in the boredom of confinement. Criminal justice agencies then use drug-positive results to note which drugs are gaining popularity, which are becoming less popular, and what types of drugs may be new to their jurisdiction. From this data, excellent planning can be done to accommodate the special needs of these particular drug users in the correctional system.

> Criminal justice agencies then use drug-positive results to note which drugs are gaining popularity, which are becoming less popular, and what types of drugs may be new to their jurisdiction. From this data, excellent planning can be done.

As an example of how criminal justice agencies can use epidemiological studies to help prepare to handle drug-positive persons appropriately, consider the rise in heroin use. As the quality of heroin has improved, smoking heroin has become more popular, especially among younger adults who would have otherwise shunned heroin use because of a fear of needles. A drug-testing program can uncover this trend in a local jurisdiction and can then help agency planners anticipate that an increasing number of people will need detoxification, methadone treatment, and other drug-abuse treatment services directed specifically toward the heroin addict.

Drug Testing Detainees/Arrestees

Drug testing can play an important information-gathering role when people are first arrested or detained for a crime. Sometimes it can even play a lifesaving role, as illustrated by this story:

> Elizabeth, a twenty-two-year-old woman, is placed under arrest by a local law-enforcement officer at 10:02 P.M. for public intoxication and indecency. She is transported by the officer to the local county jail and arrives at 10:45 P.M.

Corrections officers begin the intake process by conducting a search, during which time she is unable to stand unassisted and slumps to the floor. Corrections staff assist her to her feet and complete the search while other officers assist by holding her up. She begins shouting loudly to the more than two hundred other arrestees in the booking area that she is being raped and turns and attempts to hit the officers holding her up. She is then held down and subdued by the officers. When Elizabeth agrees to be compliant, she is escorted to a nearby chair and told to wait there until the booking process begins with a medical assessment.

After about twenty minutes, and before her medical assessment can begin, her voice rises above the din of the waiting room attracting the attention of several corrections officers who approach her. As they approach, she begins screaming and jumps to her feet and scrambles up on her chair. The officers converge on her, lift her off the chair, and gently pull her down as she continues to scream incoherently. Officers ask for her cooperation, but she does not respond to them and continues to yell. The officers move quickly to confine her in an isolation cell with a glass front so that they can continue to monitor her behavior. The confinement seems to work because she eventually becomes exhausted from pounding on the glass and sits down on the floor. Sometime after midnight, she appears to fall asleep. At 2:00 A.M., a corrections officer enters the cell and attempts to wake her to return her to the general waiting room population. She is in a sitting position on the floor with her back against the wall and her head slumped forward on her chest. She is nonresponsive. Medical staff is called. They determine that Elizabeth died in her cell. An autopsy later reveals that she died of an overdose of several drugs, including cocaine, heroin, and alcohol.

This story suggests that a drug test might have saved Elizabeth's life. Drug and alcohol screening tests can be offered to all arrestees within the medical assessment stage of jail booking facilities. This could include an offer to immediately test all those individuals who appear to be under the influence of drugs or alcohol at intake. Such a drug- and alcohol-testing program may one day become compulsory, as was suggested by President Bill Clinton in his 1996 Directive on Drug Testing Federal Arrestees. However, even in the absence of a compulsory program, jurisdictions that have offered such tests to arrestees on a voluntary basis have seen cooperation rates in excess of 80 percent. In the case of Elizabeth, her uncooperative behavior would have made such a test difficult, but not impossible. In this case, drug-testing devices such as an oral-fluids test would have permitted the medical staff person working with the corrections officers to swab Elizabeth's mouth quickly during the time she sat quietly in the chair or on the floor of the isolation cell. Such a simple test could have changed the outcome of this unfortunate situation, as Elizabeth would have been placed under more intensive supervision and perhaps even transported to a local hospital.

With encouragement from the federal government dating back to the 1980s, many jurisdictions have adopted this type of pretrial drug testing of arrestees.

Conducting a drug test as part of a medical assessment at booking or intake is also beneficial in identifying other recent drug use. Elizabeth was arrested for public intoxication since the arresting officer smelled alcohol on her breath and she did not pass a field sobriety test. However, the autopsy found she was positive not only for the drug on her arrest report (alcohol), but also for other drugs (cocaine and heroin). Using a multipanel drug test would reveal hidden drugs that an arrestee may fail to disclose on a self-report. Testing for multiple drugs provides more information that can trigger specific protocols being used to handle detainees that will ultimately lead to better outcomes for the arrestees. Table 1 gives an overview of the tests that could be done during the medical assessment phase of the booking procedure.

> Drug and alcohol screening tests can be offered to all arrestees within the medical assessment stage of jail booking facilities.

> Conducting a drug test as part of a medical assessment at booking or intake is also beneficial in identifying other recent drug use.

TABLE 1

Choosing a Drug Test for a Medical Assessment Evaluation in a Correctional Setting		
Type of Test	**Length of Drug Use Measured (Drug-Detection Window)**	**Pros and Cons**
Urine Test	Can identify drug use in the prior one to three days.	In most cases, this is the standard drug test used. It can identify a broad range of drugs and is the lowest in cost. It can be used on-site for immediate results.
Oral-Fluids Test	Can identify drug use in the prior twenty-four hours.	This is the best choice if there is concern about cheating. It can be used on-site for immediate results.
Hair Test	Can identify drug use in the prior ninety days minus the seven days immediately before the sample collection.	Although this test is more expensive, it is highly resistant to cheating. It provides rough quantitative levels of specific drug use during the ninety days before collection. It is currently not available for use on-site; results are available in several days.

There are many scenarios in which drug testing can help medical staff at a jail better grasp what is going on with an arrestee. In the criminal justice system, offenders have good reason to avoid drug- or alcohol-use detection. However, this information is critical to determining the best way to proceed with a person's arrest and conviction.

Drug Testing during Postarrest/Pretrial

Once under the control of the criminal justice system, persons are subject to testing at almost all status transition points. The DUF/ADAM system tested them at the earliest possible point— immediately after arrest and prior to any formal charge or even a first appearance or hearing on the legality of the arrest. However, bear in mind that in DUF/ADAM, the testing is voluntary, anonymous, and without consequence for any individual. Once the person has entered the system to the point of appearance before a judge, any drug testing that occurs is usually consequential.

Pretrial testing is important because the drug status of an individual under arrest may be an important consideration in deciding whether or not to release someone before further legal processing. After the determination of the legality of the arrest, the court must determine the appropriate course of action for the person who is now in legal custody. Since drug use is tied to criminal conduct, the court must evaluate the likelihood that the arrestee will engage in criminal conduct while waiting for his or her court appearance. Drug use is one of several factors that the court can weigh in making that determination.

Drug testing at this stage occurs prior to the appearance for pretrial release, and the outcome of the test is one of the factors the court considers regarding release and its conditions. Drug testing can also take place after the hearing to determine whether, during release, the person needs to undergo continued testing or perhaps be referred to drug treatment.

The court has the legal authority to impose conditions on the detained citizen in order to ensure the arrestee appears in court to answer for any charges and to protect the public from further harm by the defendant. The arrestee, under the court's consideration for postarrest release back into the community, can be required to abide by certain conditions imposed by the court. These conditions include maintaining a known place of residence, abiding by restrictions on the degree of travel and regulation of social contacts while under supervision, maintaining contact with the supervising agency, and honoring the condition of remaining drug abstinent if he or she is a drug user or has tested drug positive as a pretrial detainee. The condition of drug abstinence includes a requirement to report for periodic drug testing to assure the court that abstinence is indeed being maintained. A failure to maintain drug abstinence will trigger sanctions.

Traditionally, pretrial services (like almost all other programs using drug tests within the criminal justice system) have relied on urinalysis. We will discuss the technical details of the various methods

> Drug testing can also take place after the hearing to determine whether, during release, the person needs to undergo continued testing or perhaps be referred to drug treatment.

of testing for drugs in chapter 4, but we need at this point to consider briefly the operational consequences of using particular drug-testing technology.

While urinalysis is well established, relatively inexpensive, and the oldest of all the currently used techniques, it has some important limitations. The most serious of these is the relatively short retrospective "time window" for detecting past use of many of the most commonly abused illicit drugs. For cocaine, heroin, and amphetamine, for example, urinalysis is largely ineffective as a detector after forty-eight to seventy-two hours have passed since the last drug use. This constrains the interpretation of urinalysis-based drug testing as a valid indicator of drug abstinence.

The consequence of this limitation has been addressed in two ways. One is to utilize a randomized testing schedule to thwart anticipation of a testing date. Another is to utilize a different type of test—often referred to as "alternative matrices." These have primarily been of two types—analysis of sweat patches and hair samples. Both of these can offer a longer retrospective window, so they can limit or reduce the concern with evasion through manipulation of the timing of the drug test.

Diversion Programs

When offenders are arrested and taken into custody by the police, several outcomes are possible. One is that the detainee may be released without charge. A second is that the detainee may be charged with a crime. If this second course unfolds for the detainee, he or she is likely to face several possibilities as a consequence of facing criminal charges. One is to take the case before a court for trial and a consequent verdict. Oftentimes, however, persons charged with a criminal offense may have several other options that are offered to them in lieu of going into a courtroom. These alternatives can be grouped together under the term *diversion*. By diversion, we mean that the individual is directed onto an alternative pathway to resolve his or her criminal case. Most important, the defendant in the criminal case has options to resolve the charges without having to

By diversion, we mean that the individual is directed onto an alternative pathway to resolve his or her criminal case.

go to trial. Diversion programs, if they are successfully completed, typically result in a dismissal of the original criminal case.

Diversion is not offered to all defendants. Cases involving violence, nondrug felony offenses, repeated offenses, meaningful criminal history, or similar factors are usually excluded. All diversion programs are local, and therefore the standards and practices vary from jurisdiction to jurisdiction. Most diversion programs include an assessment of the social and psychological characteristics of the offender and make varying efforts to help improve the life circumstances of the offender, thus lessening the chances of future criminal behavior.

Drug testing can help assess the individual's drug usage, which may indicate a need for drug treatment while in a diversion program. Drug testing can also be used as a monitoring tool during a diversion program.

Drug Courts

Another approach to diversion, but one that occurs at the judicial rather than prosecutorial stage is the *drug court*. The drug court assumes the responsibility of supervising and monitoring an offender who has been charged with a drug crime but is not likely to go to trial. As with the earlier form of prosecutorial diversion, this situation usually applies to persons and situations where the basic facts of the case are not in dispute—the person does not intend to deny possession and/or use of an illicit drug. Rather, other circumstances such as the nature of the offense, the criminal record (or often the lack of criminal record), and similar considerations lead to a decision to offer the offender the opportunity to transit through the sanctioning phase of the process with less damage to his or her future than would be the case if proceeding to a conventional criminal court and pleading guilty.

> Drug courts handle substance-abusing offenders, usually persons who are charged with simple possession or various "under the influence" violations.

Drug courts handle substance-abusing offenders, usually persons who are charged with simple possession or various "under the influence" violations. For the most part, the court handles offenders who are nonviolent (and typically lack a violent history), offenders who are not involved in drug distribution, and offenders who are abusers of substances both licit (such as alcohol) and illicit. For most of these persons, their dependence on and abuse of psychoactive drugs is one of the root causes of their legal problems. Drug courts rely upon coordination of many different components of the criminal justice system as well as community agencies. In addition to the judiciary and the office of the prosecutor, they use input from experts in the areas of mental health, social service, and substance-abuse treatment. The fundamental objective of the drug court is intervention to break the cycle of substance abuse, addiction, and crime.

The first step in the drug court process is to identify the appropriate offenders. Drug testing is an important first step in the drug court process, as it is in all diversion programs. Drug testing identifies unambiguously the nature of the drug or drugs involved. Offenders who are admitted to a drug court are generally put through an assessment that identifies not only the particulars of their substance abuse problems, but also allows for an examination of the nature of related problems, such as health, family, psychological, and skill deficiencies. Once a determination and assessment is complete, then the court is able to act by placing the offender in appropriate treatment, rehabilitation, and similar programs as the assessment process warrants.

> Drug testing identifies unambiguously the nature of the drug or drugs involved.

Drug courts do carry out sanctions. The treatment of offenders, while aimed at rehabilitation and recovery, is also rigorous in monitoring the offender's behavior under the court's control. The drug court carries out a variety of monitoring functions under what may be generally called "community supervision." Under the control of the presiding judge, the offenders experience an intense regimen of case management, drug testing, and probationary supervision, including regularly scheduled status hearings, before the court's judge.

Generally, drug courts offer four fundamental improvements to traditional criminal case processing: they decrease recidivism, save money, increase retention in treatment, and provide affordable treatment.

Drug Testing during Postconviction Release: Probation, House Arrest, and Similar Programs

Another setting for drug testing within the criminal justice system is the monitoring of postconviction offenders who are sentenced to some custodial status that keeps them in the community and out of a prison or jail. This can be generally called *postconviction drug testing*. It differs from the drug court and related diversion programs in that these individuals are convicted of an offense in a criminal court and are sentenced for their offense. Typically, they are permitted to serve this sentence within a released setting. However, if they fail to conform to the conditions of the court, they can be required to serve the remainder of the sentence in a correctional institution.

No other segment of the criminal justice population approaches the number of offenders who are convicted of an offense and serve their sentence within some community setting. Of the approximately 6.8 million persons in the United States under some type of correctional supervision, roughly 4.8 million are either on probationary status or are parolees. Twenty-five percent of all probationers are drug-law offenders, and an additional 17 percent are driving-while-intoxicated offenders. Based on survey research, more than 80 percent of these persons have a history of drug use, and more than 65 percent report having used drugs regularly during their lives. More than half were current drug users at the time of the commission of the offense for which they are serving their sentence, and one-third of them self-report being drug intoxicated when they were actually in the process of committing the offense for which they were convicted.

Persons convicted of an offense who are not sentenced to a period of incarceration are almost universally placed under a probationary or similar correctional supervisory status (often called "house arrest" or "community supervision"). These individuals remain in the community, but they operate under varying conditions and typically have restrictions on their liberty. In fact, more than 98 percent of offenders sentenced to a probationary status have conditions imposed on their release back into the community. Approximately 40 percent of them

> Twenty-five percent of all probationers are drug-law offenders, and an additional 17 percent are driving-while-intoxicated offenders.

are required to remain drug- (and in some cases alcohol-) abstinent. Of these 40 percent, more than 30 percent face mandatory drug testing. Typically, these programs use urine that is collected under the supervision of an officer, which is then sent to a local laboratory for analysis. Drug- and/or alcohol-abuse treatment is almost always a mandated condition of release.

The protocol of postconviction drug testing, while for the most part universally accepted and practiced, is quite variable in its application. The intensity of testing may vary widely, ranging from frequent, random screenings to testing that is only done on suspicion. The response to a positive test can also vary widely, from doing nothing other than issuing an informal warning to giving a referral to treatment to seeking a revocation of community placement and returning the individual to institutional incarceration. The most frequent response is to increase the frequency of drug testing, with a threat that repeated positives will generate a potential revocation of probation.

As the following story illustrates, postconviction drug testing can simplify the parole process and alleviate some of the struggles that parole officers deal with on a daily basis:

> Tom arrives at his probation office for his monthly meeting. He signs in at the front desk and waits calmly for his probation officer to call him in. After about five minutes, his probation officer comes into the waiting room carrying a plastic cup with a screw-type lid. Since Tom has been through this exercise many times, he and his probation officer make small talk as they head into the restroom at the end of the hall. Tom takes the cup and begins to urinate into it, while the probation officer sits in an adjoining stall with a one-way mirror so that he can directly observe that the urine is coming from Tom and has not been smuggled in, diluted, or adulterated. Tom screws on the lid, and then both men leave their stalls and the probation officer asks Tom to put his signature on the cup. The cup is placed into

The protocol of postconviction drug testing, while for the most part universally accepted and practiced, is quite variable in its application.

a plastic bag that is signed and dated to preserve the legal chain of custody. The probation officer and Tom enter the office where they review last month's negative drug-test results and discuss specific questions about Tom's employment and personal life. The probation officer then asks Tom if he may cut a few strands of hair from Tom's head since he is interested in comparing the results of a hair test to those of the urine test. Tom reluctantly agrees.

In a few days, the results come back to the probation officer that the urine sample is negative for the five specific drugs in the test panel. The results also come back from the hair test, and the probation officer notes that Tom has a moderate level of cocaine in his hair. When confronted with these results at their next scheduled monthly meeting, Tom admits that he sometimes used cocaine, especially on weekends, but always stopped about three days before coming in to their scheduled meeting. The probation officer informs Tom that he can no longer game the system that way. His illegal drug use must stop, or he will be arrested and sent back to the judge with a recommendation for his incarceration at a correctional facility. Tom is shaken. His next two monthly hair specimens are analyzed only for the length of hair closest to his head. In both the hair sample and the urine sample, the results are negative. The probation officer now knows that Tom is making progress and feels for the first time that as a probation officer, he is not just wasting his time testing street-smart offenders gaming the system.

Drug tests are valuable additions to probation, parole, and community-release programs because they can provide law enforcement and the courts with critical information about the true nature of an offender's drug use. However, as the scenario above demonstrates, there are specific limitations to each type of drug test that can sometimes be used by offenders to their advantage. We will discuss those limitations in the next chapter.

In some jurisdictions, Intensive Supervision Probation (ISP) is used so that probation officers are relieved of much of their caseload and instead work more closely with each offender. One of the concerns about such programs is the use of intensive urine drug testing (every few days), which takes an enormous amount of officers' time and is very expensive. Again, drug testing the hair of a probationer may solve this dilemma, since only one sample needs to be taken to cover an entire month rather than the ten samples of urine that would otherwise have to be collected to cover the same amount of time.

Drug Testing the Incarcerated Offender

Another group to consider for drug testing comprises those persons who have been convicted of a criminal offense and who are sentenced to a period of confinement in prison or in jail. More than two million persons are currently incarcerated in prisons or jails in the United States. About two-thirds of these offenders are held in federal and state prisons, and about one-third are held in local jails. A substantial number of these individuals are incarcerated for drug crimes— 60 percent of federal inmates, 21 percent of state inmates, and 26 percent of jail inmates. About 80 percent of them have a history of drug abuse, and about two-thirds of them have a history of regular drug use.

Drug testing is conducted on a substantial proportion of prison and jail inmates, but it is not universally used in all incarceration facilities. According to the Bureau of Justice Statistics, about 30 percent of institutions do not report any formal drug-testing protocol. Those institutions that do utilize a regular testing regimen, or have a formally established protocol for drug testing, are most likely to test on "indication of use." About 70 percent of institutions reported this criterion. It is usually triggered by either behavior that appears consistent with intoxication or the discovery and seizure of illicit drugs within the institution. Roughly half of the institutions have a

> Another group to consider for drug testing comprises those persons who have been convicted of a criminal offense and who are sentenced to a period of confinement in prison or in jail.

random testing system in place, and a smaller percentage (about 30 percent) utilize some additional criteria, such as a return to the institution from some other locale (e.g., furloughs or relocation due to legal proceedings). Only about 5 percent reported universally testing all inmates at admission to the facility.

If an inmate tests positive for one or more illicit drugs, he or she typically faces a variety of sanctions. The sanctions are divided into administrative and legal responses. The most common administrative response is that the inmate will experience a loss of some privileges within the system, such as phone access, library privileges, or similar nonentitled activities. Additionally or optionally, the inmates also face such administrative punishments as loss of earned "good time," being reclassified into a more strictly monitored security level, and going into isolation/separation. On a legal level, the inmate can be charged with a crime (e.g., possession of a controlled substance). This can result in additional time being added to the inmate's original sentence.

Drug Testing Correctional Employees

One final way in which drug testing is used in a correctional setting, as it is in many other employment settings, is to screen applicants as well as to monitor law-enforcement officers and other criminal justice system employees to assure the public that policing and correctional agencies operate "drug free." This purpose for drug testing will not be addressed in great detail in this manual. For appropriate employment drug-testing protocol, it is recommended that a correctional facility contact a large, local employer to understand its drug-testing procedures and practices.

4

■　■　■　■　■

An Overview of
Drug-Testing Technologies

What Is Drug Testing?

Drug testing means using specialized instruments and chemical techniques to identify the presence of a drug or a drug metabolite through testing some type of biological specimen collected from an individual. From this information, a person such as a caseworker, a medical review officer, or a corrections officer evaluates the drug-using status of the person undergoing assessment. The specimen type is often referred to as a "test matrix."

What Type of Specimen Should Be Collected?

The first step of any drug-testing protocol in a criminal justice setting is to take an appropriate biological sample. What's appropriate is not as straight-forward as it might seem, as a host of factors need to be considered, including the following:

- the initial expense of the drug test

- the degree of intrusion on a person's privacy

- the risk of cheating

- the specification of a quantitative or qualitative (positive or negative only) result and the length of time being studied

- the degree of convenience of collecting, handling, and storing the specimen

- the degree of acceptable risk in handling potentially infectious body fluids

We will cover each of these considerations briefly in the following pages, and later in this chapter we will pay particular attention to the cost-benefit ratio of the various tests and biological samples.

Initial Expense

The initial expense of a drug test varies widely. There are several reasons for this: (1) Some technologies are inherently more expensive to implement because of the nature of the testing materials or hazardous (even radioactive) wastes they produce; (2) some alternatives will include tests for one, several, or sometimes many drugs for one price and from one biological sample; and (3) some tests involve the use of labor-intensive laboratory equipment by highly paid and specially trained laboratory personnel as opposed to the use of high-speed, automated laboratory machines or even on-site testing used by others. For example, the initial cost of doing a urine test would be about $10 for a five-drug screen at a high-volume laboratory that uses immunoassay tests and is local to the correctional facility (so that shipping samples is not required); the initial costs of an oral-fluids test to cover a six-drug screen at a laboratory that would receive specimens by mail would be about $11; and the initial costs of a hair test for a five-drug screen where the specimen is sent by mail to a specialized laboratory is about $40.

Degree of Intrusion

One factor to consider when deciding which biological sample to collect is the degree to which collecting the sample is intrusive. When a urine sample is collected, for example, many correctional facilities directly observe the process to ensure that the person being tested doesn't use a "clean" person's urine in place of his or her own. Careful and direct observation of the sample collection is critical to preserve the validity of the drug test, but direct observation makes urine testing an extremely intrusive process. Collecting saliva and sweat is much less intrusive because these methods involve swabbing the inside of the mouth with a cotton-tipped stick or placing a patch on a small section of skin. Even less intrusive is collecting a small sample of hair (about forty strands) from the head.

> The initial expense of a drug test varies widely.

> One factor to consider when deciding which biological sample to collect is the degree to which collecting the sample is intrusive.

Risk of Cheating

The degree to which the justice system is willing to tolerate cheating on tests is another consideration when deciding which test to use. In a correctional setting, arrestees being tested often try to hide the true extent of their current substance use. Urine samples are especially vulnerable to cheating. In fact, an entire industry has grown up around cheating on the urine test. Clean urine can be purchased by anyone in head shops that sell drug paraphernalia. In addition, chemical adulterants, which are sold in these same stores and over the Internet, claim to be able to foul up any subsequent chemical analysis. Adulterants are either dropped into the sample while a person urinates into it or taken orally some hours before a test.

The potential to cheat with a hair, saliva, or sweat sample is relatively low. Some head shops now sell clean saliva samples, but it is difficult for people to substitute that saliva for their own if normal testing procedures are followed. Advertisements have appeared that also claim to sell hair-cleansing products that remove all traces of drugs; however, these products have been found to be ineffective. In fact, short of completely dissolving the hair, the drugs are trapped in the hair virtually forever. The drugs were laid down in the hair when it was produced in the hair follicle. For more in-depth information on the issue of cheating, see chapter 6.

> The degree to which the justice system is willing to tolerate cheating on tests is another consideration when deciding which test to use.

Quantitative versus Qualitative

Another major factor to consider is the extent to which you wish to have a quantitative assessment of drugs detected in the analysis. That is, do you want to try to estimate the *amount* (a *quantitative* analysis) of drug used as well as the *type* (a *qualitative* analysis) of drug used?

A quantitative result showing the exact concentration of drugs in the body is rarely reported, except in forensic or autopsy settings. In correctional settings, results are usually reported in a simple qualitative fashion as either positive or negative at specified cutoff levels. The advantage to the correctional facility is that the task of interpreting these drug-test results is simplified somewhat because the threshold has already been determined. These thresholds, or cutoff levels, are specified by governmental agencies for federally mandated drug tests and then adopted by many testing laboratories so that the trivial incidental exposure to minute amounts of drugs in our environment can never be confused with actual drug use. One example of such incidental exposure is U.S. paper currency, most of which has been contaminated with trace amounts of cocaine. The thresholds are set high enough, however, that even a person who works with money all day, such as a bank teller, would never be mistaken as a drug user. These thresholds are identified as specific quantities so that the automated machines that are typically used to test samples of urine, saliva, sweat, and hair are simply calibrated to register a "positive" if this predetermined threshold has been exceeded or a "negative" if it has not been exceeded. That way, there is no numeric or quantitative record of the result of these types of drug tests, since only the qualitative nature of the result is reported.

This lack of a quantitative result is initially confusing to people who are used to thinking of alcohol testing, where quantitative levels below certain standards are considered to be acceptable for driving and for other activities, but higher levels are equated with intoxication. In contrast to alcohol testing, there is no correlation for drug testing (other than blood testing) between levels of impairment or intoxication and quantitative levels of the identified drugs. In addition, unlike alcohol, there is no legal use of the drugs usually tested for, such as cocaine, marijuana, and heroin. The relevant information from drug tests used in correctional settings is not the *level* of the drug identified, but the *presence* of the drug, since it is the use itself that is illegal.

> The relevant information from drug tests used in correctional settings is not the *level* of the drug identified, but the *presence* of the drug, since it is the use itself that is illegal.

Samples of urine, saliva, and sweat all typically provide qualitative, yes-no results. In some correctional cases, it is beneficial to have what is called semiquantitative results. Hair samples fall into this category because the results are not only coded as positive or negative, but they also reveal the relative amounts of drugs found. In most cases, this means that results are reported according to the level of use, ranging from Level 1 use (consistent with relatively low drug use) to Level 5 use (corresponding to a high level of use of the identified drug). Even if urine is quantitatively tested, there is little, if any, relationship between the levels of drugs in urine and the extent of drug use. One of the biggest determinants of the concentration of drugs in urine is the amount of fluid consumed in the hour or two before the test. Semiquantitative hair-test results are correlated with levels of drug use within the past ninety days. The more extensive semiquantitative information from a hair test is particularly useful at intake into a correctional setting because treatment decisions are often determined by this estimate of the intensity of drug use.

Length of Detection

Because drugs distribute themselves into different fluids and tissues in the body, the selection of a specimen type automatically imposes a "time window" associated with that specimen. In other words, the particular time period—called the retrospective period—varies depending on the choice of specimen. From the time drugs are ingested until they are excreted, they are involved in a dynamic process of change. Different specimens reflect different stages of this dynamic process. For example, consider a hypothetical drug abuser who primarily smokes crack cocaine.

> Because drugs distribute themselves into different fluids and tissues in the body, the selection of a specimen type automatically imposes a "time window" associated with that specimen.

Crack cocaine, delivered to the surface of the lungs, quickly moves in large concentrations into blood plasma. Indeed, the rapidity of absorption through the alveoli is very similar to intravenous injection. Thus a blood sample harvested just a few minutes after a person smokes crack will have cocaine present in it. It will take twenty to thirty minutes for appreciable amounts of cocaine or cocaine metabolite to appear in the urine. And after cocaine is no longer in the circulating blood plasma, it will still be present in the urine stored in the bladder. Thus blood and urine have different time windows. The current technology that offers the longest retrospective time window (the one that "looks back" the longest) is hair analysis. While it will take three to five days for cocaine to appear in the hair of a cocaine user, the cocaine appears "locked" into the hair virtually permanently.

Unless the hair is removed or dissolved, the cocaine will be detectable, even months after the ingestion of the drug. This includes both scalp and body hair. The same long-term presence is true for fingernails and toenails.

Convenience and Safety

Finally, the convenience of storing and handling the specimens, including the degree of risk of infectious disease transmission by contact with body fluids, needs to be considered. By now, everyone in a correctional setting has probably been trained to deal safely with body fluids. People working in criminal justice programs are well aware of the risks associated with accidental contact, especially with blood. Urine, saliva, and sweat must be treated as potentially risky body fluids as well. Collectors and handlers of these specimens should wear protective equipment, including gloves and face shields. Hair is the only specimen used for drug testing that can be collected without concern for disease transmission.

Table 2 is a synopsis of the relative performance and other practical features of the various specimen types used in drug testing. Here is a brief description of each characteristic outlined in the table:

- *Expense:* cost of the test
- *Intrusion:* the degree to which the specimen collection is intrusive
- *Retrospection:* the period of time for which the specimen can reveal past use
- *Evasion:* the level of ease or difficulty for a person attempting to evade or cheat on the test
- *Quantitation:* the ability of the test to offer some estimate of the extent or intensity of drug use
- *Convenience of storage/handling:* the level of ease or difficulty for handling the specimen
- *Risk for infectious disease:* the degree to which the specimen may be a biohazard

> The convenience of storing and handling the specimens, including the degree of risk of infectious disease transmission by contact with body fluids, needs to be considered.

TABLE 2

A Comparison of Drug-Test Sample Types				
Sample Characteristics	**Sample Type**			
	Urine	*Hair*	*Saliva*	*Sweat*
Expense	Low	High	Moderate	Moderate
Intrusion	High	Low	Moderate	Moderate
Retrospection	Low	High	Low	High*
Evasion	High	Low	Unknown	Low
Quantitation	No	Semi-	No	No
Convenience of Storage/Handling	Low	High	Low	Moderate
Risk for Infectious Disease	Low	Very low	Low	Very low

* Sweat-patch testing looks forward from the time the patch is applied (this is the only test that does), but it looks back from the time the patch is removed to be analyzed. The window of detection for a sweat patch is the period of time that it is worn. Thus, the window of detection for sweat patches is longer than for urine or oral fluids.

Screening Tests

Drug testing is the chemical identification of the presence of a drug of abuse in a biological specimen—a toxicological analysis. The chemical processes used in drug tests may identify either the parent drug, such as cocaine, or the parent drug's principal metabolite, which for cocaine is benzoylecgonine. Metabolites, which are produced principally in the liver, are often present in higher concentrations and for longer periods of time than the parent drug, so they are often the chemicals identified, especially for marijuana, cocaine, and heroin.

Specimen testing is typically divided into two steps. First, a screening test indicates whether certain drugs are present in the sample. If the screening test is positive, a confirmatory test is conducted to determine precisely which drug or drugs are present. The laboratory can apply one of two types of screening technologies to the biological specimen submitted for drug testing: *thin-layer chromatography* or *immunoassays*. Either of these two laboratory tests can be used for any type of specimen, whether urine, hair, oral fluids, or sweat. Both types of tests are equally precise in their drug identification. The choice of sample is not an issue of accuracy but a matter of the many factors described earlier. Although the laboratory will need to prepare the samples differently (hair is a solid and must be dissolved before it can be analyzed like the other specimens), the chemistry of the analytical procedure itself, and therefore the final accuracy of the result that is based on this science, is always the same.

Blood is rarely used to test for drugs of abuse (except in death investigations), not because the drugs are not there but because it is relatively difficult to obtain a blood sample and prepare it for testing. As a result, blood testing for drugs of abuse is much more expensive than is testing of the other types of samples. Immunoassays are typically chosen for use since thin-layer chromatography is labor intensive, while immunoassay techniques lend themselves to high-speed automated processes and can even be utilized in on-site field-test kits. It is helpful, however, to understand the technology behind both the thin-layer chromatography tests and immunoassay tests, as well as the lesser-used ion scan technology.

Thin-Layer Chromatography (TLC)

One of the original laboratory-based toxicological tests for drugs of abuse involves the use of thin-layer chromatography (TLC). This process begins by separating the components of a mixture. The principle behind this technique is fairly simple. When a person gets a drop of spaghetti sauce on his or her clothes, the drop begins to spread out over the cloth. After a while, the spot shows up with rings of different colors around it. The chunk of tomato is at the center, surrounded by some heavy oil, which is surrounded by some lighter oils and finally a ring of water. The color rings correspond

> Specimen testing is typically divided into two steps. First, a screening test indicates whether certain drugs are present in the sample. If the screening test is positive, a confirmatory test is conducted to determine precisely which drug or drugs are present.

to the "chroma" or "color" in chromatography. The heavier substances move the shortest distance and the most slowly. The lightest substances move the farthest and the fastest. Basically, what we have in TLC is a technology reflected in sloppy eating.

In the laboratory, a small amount of the liquid specimen is placed on a thin layer of glass coated with a special granular material made up of silica or alumina. The plate is turned on its end, vertically, with the bottom dipped into a bath of special solvent. The solvent begins to travel slowly up the coating through capillary action, like water on the cuff of one's pants hanging in a puddle. Over time, the whole leg gets soaked. As the solvent moves up, it takes some of the specimen with it, with the lightest components of the specimen traveling farthest up the coated glass. Unlike the spaghetti stain, however, this stain won't be visible to the naked eye because the components are generally clear. But when the lab technician shines an ultraviolet light on them, they show as streaks of fluorescence—bright spots on a dark background. Sometimes a chemical dye is sprayed over the entire coated glass plate, and then the lab technician simply watches as colored spots appear. These spots are then compared to standards that are kept on file. When a match is found, the drugs are identified.

Thin-layer chromatography takes very little time overall and is very effective at finding exceedingly small amounts of drugs in just a few drops of liquid. It has three disadvantages compared to immunoassay-screening drug tests, however: it is labor intensive and cannot be automated since it requires highly trained laboratory personnel to interpret the results; it does not produce quantitative results; and since the fluid continues to move across the surface of the test plate, the results are not fixed, or permanent, but continue to change over time, making preservation of the original evidence impossible. One advantage of TLC over the immunoassay is that a single test can identify many different drugs, while the immunoassay is specific for each drug tested. When looking for many drugs in a single sample, it can be less expensive to use TLC.

One advantage of TLC over the immunoassay is that a single test can identify many different drugs, while the immunoassay is specific for each drug tested. When looking for many drugs in a single sample, it can be less expensive to use TLC.

Immunoassay

Drug tests based on immunoassay techniques are far more prevalent in today's laboratories because they are fast, they are inexpensive, and the entire process can be automated with machines capable of testing hundreds of samples per hour. The immunoassay-screening drug-test analysis is based on the mammalian body's immune system, which uses antibodies to both identify and destroy invading pathogens. In the case of laboratory-based drug tests, antibodies are created in a laboratory, not taken from humans. Each antibody is designed to locate only one foreign substance—the specific molecule of the drug being tested for. The antibody ignores everything but the drug because nothing else will fit its molecular pattern, just as a key fits into only one lock.

As soon as the antibody finds a molecule of that drug, it latches onto it in the same way the human body's antibodies latch onto pathogens. In the body, this process disables, destroys, and signals disposal for the offending foreign substance. In the laboratory, antibodies are instead linked to a specially designed signal, such as an enzyme, a radioisotope, or a fluorescent dye. When a drop of this specially designed immunoassay antibody solution is put into a vial containing a small amount of urine or other bodily fluid sample, the antibodies attach themselves to the molecules of that drug. The solution is then tested for the presence of these signals, and if they are found, there is an indication of the presence of that drug. For example, the vials of urine mixed with antibodies and signal substances can be passed in front of an ultraviolet light source by a machine at a very high rate of speed. If the machine detects that the sample fluoresces, the drug of interest is present. Then, in a manner similar to thin-layer chromatography drug tests, the results are reported as positive or negative for that particular drug in that specific sample.

The chief problem with immunoassays concerns cross-reactivity, where, in some cases, a test will indicate that a positive result has been found for an illegal drug, when in fact the individual has only

> The chief problem with immunoassays concerns cross-reactivity, where, in some cases, a test will indicate that a positive result has been found for an illegal drug, when in fact the individual has only consumed some over-the-counter medication.

consumed some over-the-counter medication. Although this is a fairly rare occurrence, and the manufacturers of immunoassay technologies work very hard to prevent such reactions, such results are possible. While this sounds dire, this actually has become the springboard from which the two-step testing process that involves a confirmatory analysis was founded.

Ion Scans

Ion scans are a relatively new addition to on-site drug detection. Recent air travelers have experienced this new technology first-hand, as it is now used in many airports to screen passengers and their luggage for molecules associated with explosives and drugs of abuse. The ion scan device is about the size of a microwave oven with a small hose similar to one on a vacuum cleaner. A technician places a gauze pad over the nozzle of the hose and brushes it over the clothing, hair, and skin of the person who he or she wishes to test. Particles of drugs that have attached themselves to these surfaces are collected onto the gauze pad, which is then introduced directly into the ion scan machine. The machine can simultaneously test for thousands of substances within seconds, automatically providing a "green-light" or "red-light" indication of a person's status.

> Ion scans are a relatively new addition to on-site drug detection.

People who produce red lights are confronted with the results in order to promote honesty. While potentially useful, ion scans are initially expensive and require a very high-level technician to maintain them properly, as the devices are very sensitive. The proper action after a positive ion scan test result is to interview the person testing positive and to proceed with specific drug testing to confirm or refute the ion scan result. Sanctions should not be imposed from a positive ion scan without either an admission of guilt or a positive drug-test result because exposure to drugs may occur innocently in the contemporary environment. Ion scans are not a common testing method used in correctional settings at this time.

Confirmatory Tests

As mentioned earlier, a potential problem with screening tests is cross-reactivity. In some cases, an immunoassay test may react with a number of compounds that are very similar to the drug it's trying to find. For example, if an individual took a prescription drug such as hydrocodone (Vicodin) under the care of a dentist, the screening test may show that this person tests positive for opiates even though hydrocodone is not an illegal opiate. A confirmatory test uses a different technology to confirm exactly which drug the screening test is identifying. The high degree of specificity in the confirming test is expensive and so is conducted only when an inexpensive screening test has shown a positive result and when it is important to rule out cross-reactivity.

The gold standard of toxicological drug testing that is used for confirmatory drug tests is *gas chromatography / mass spectrometry,* or *GC/MS*. This is strictly a laboratory device, operated by highly trained chemists. It is capable of determining the exact makeup of specific molecules within a tested sample. Here there is no cross-reactivity. GC/MS technology is one of the most powerful analytical instruments on the planet and, in addition to verifying drug tests, it is used to identify any unknown substance.

> The gold standard of toxicological drug testing that is used for confirmatory drug tests is *gas chromatography/ mass spectrometry, or GC/MS.*

The GC/MS procedure can be broken into two distinct processes. Here we give a simplified description of a complex and rapidly evolving scientific process. First, it is necessary to break apart the mixture of substances present in the sample. Just as with the spaghetti stain mentioned earlier, some substances travel faster than other substances. In GC/MS, instead of liquids passing across cloth or over a coated glass plate, vapors are allowed to flow through a long tube. The faster vapors travel down this tube ahead of slower ones. Given a long enough tube, when a biological sample is vaporized in a flame, the vapors come out of the other end of the tube in the order of their transit speeds.

With GC/MS technology, specific substances are chosen to coat the inside of the tube, or column, to slow the gases down on the basis of what is known as selective adsorption. The type of column used depends on the properties of the specimen being analyzed. To speed the flow of the sample vapors through the column, an inert carrier gas such as helium is pumped into the column at the same time.

As the vapors emerge from the end of the long column, their travel or elution time is recorded by a sensor. A graph or chromatogram is automatically made that characterizes the components of the sample as a kind of high-tech signature. That signature is used to identify many substances, including drugs, with remarkable precision. That is how the GC, or gas chromatography, part of the GC/MS test works.

The next part of the GC/MS process is mass spectrometry. In this part of the process, the sample vapors are given an electrical charge, or ionized. Then they are accelerated with the use of an internal magnetic field into a special detector. Because each ion has a different mass/charge ratio, it travels a specific and characteristic distance over the sensor, making a virtual rainbow of ions. The heavier ions travel shorter distances than the lighter ions. This rainbow, or spectrum, of ions is characteristic of specific substances. It is used to make exact identification of each substance that is being looked for. The linking of gas chromatography with mass spectrometry results in a technology with remarkable precision.

Why Do Both Screening and Confirmatory Tests?

In many situations, the screening test alone is sufficient. Most screening tests are accurate because the manufacturers of the patented antibodies work hard to get a high degree of specificity. When a person, after screening positive, admits recent drug use, there is no need to do a confirming test. When a single test result does not lead to severe consequences, such as violation of probation and a return to jail, then there may be no need to conduct a confirming test.

When, however, there are significant consequences to a particular drug-test result, such as termination from a treatment program or arrest for violation of a court order, then there may be a good reason to proceed to the confirming test because even a small chance of error is unacceptable in this situation. When particular drug-test results are highly consequential, and especially when they are disputed, it is important to retain the sample for possible future retest, either at

When there are significant consequences to a particular drug-test result, such as termination from a treatment program or arrest for violation of a court order, then there may be a good reason to proceed to the confirming test.

the correctional setting or at the drug-test laboratory, in addition to conducting a confirmatory test. Urine samples that test positive are typically preserved in a freezer for one year, while positive hair samples can be kept in a locked file cabinet indefinitely.

The smart way to run a laboratory-testing program is to test all the samples with immunoassays—the least expensive, least time-consuming, and most automated technology. When the test is positive for an illegal drug, save the remainder of the original sample for a confirmatory test later. During confirmatory testing, another small sample of liquid is withdrawn from the container. The container holding the original liquid is then frozen and kept at the confirming laboratory for an extended period of time in case there is a need to retest the original liquid for any reason—including responding to a challenge that the initial test was not properly conducted. If the screening test is negative—as most samples are—then simply discard the entire sample. No subsequent confirmatory tests need to be run on those samples.

What If the Confirmatory Test Results Do Not Agree with the Screening Test Results?

The confirmatory test always overrules the screening result because the confirming test uses a more precise technology. If, for example, a person takes a dose of an over-the-counter cold medication and then tests positive for amphetamines on a screening drug test, the GC/MS confirmation test can be used to test *specifically* for amphetamine and methamphetamine. The confirmatory test would ignore molecules found in some over-the-counter cold medications that cross-react with amphetamine and methamphetamine in immunoassay tests. If the person has only consumed the cold medication and not the illegal substance, the results of the confirmatory test are found to be negative for amphetamine or methamphetamine. Upon getting the results, the screening laboratory reports that the tested person is negative for amphetamine/methamphetamine.

A correctional setting that uses a laboratory-based screening test and routinely uses confirming tests when appropriate will always

> The confirmatory test always overrules the screening result because the confirming test uses a more precise technology.

have accurate results when the confirming test uses GC/MS or equivalent technology. In a correctional setting, where a single positive test can lead to serious consequences for the individual, the highest standard is for all positive screening results to be submitted for confirmatory testing with positive samples retained for a year for possible retesting.

What Are the Practical Considerations of the Two-Step Process?

When determining how to manage screening and confirmatory testing, correctional settings need to consider the following factors:

- the expense of conducting two tests
- the time required to obtain a result (on-site versus off-site testing)
- the time frames inherent in the different biological specimens

Expense

Conducting confirmatory testing costs more than conducting a screening test only. Remember that it is just the positive samples from the screening tests that are subsequently subjected to confirmatory testing. The first step in estimating the total program costs for the two-step process is to estimate what percentage of samples might be found positive by the screening test. If that percentage of initial positives is very low—for example, in the neighborhood of 5 percent, as might be expected when conducting testing while offenders are in a court-ordered residential treatment program— the cost to implement the two-step process may be affordable. If that percentage is estimated to be 100 percent—as might be expected at intake to a drug-court program—the confirmatory testing expense might be prohibitively expensive. In some situations, it is possible to pass the costs of confirmatory testing on to the individuals undergoing drug testing as part of their evaluation, as is sometimes done when conducting court-ordered evaluations of people arrested for DUIs.

> Conducting confirmatory testing costs more than conducting a screening test only.

Time Required to Obtain a Result

Some correctional facilities operate their own certified urine-testing laboratories for screening and are able to run urine tests inexpensively.

This is especially cost effective for large multisite correctional facilities. In this scenario, a correctional staff member picks up and delivers drug-test samples on a regular basis each day. The test results, typically available within hours, are faxed back to the individual staff members. If an outside testing laboratory is used and confirmatory tests are run routinely for positive screening tests, it may take two days for the test results to reach the correctional facility. Test results that are quickly confirmed are far more useful in correctional settings than are test results that are available after two or more days. The time required to obtain a result is a powerful argument for on-site testing, especially in large facilities.

Small correctional facilities sometimes use on-site test kits for screening. With a test kit, facilities are able to get screening results immediately, the kit is less expensive than an off-site laboratory, and the facilities can still go to an off-site laboratory for the more precise confirmatory test. With a kit, the cost of each screening test is slightly higher than it is at a high-volume, in-house drug-testing laboratory, but the tests are easily conducted by nonlaboratory personnel (usually the correctional staff member who obtained the sample). In addition, knowing the results immediately can be a critically important part of a correctional program when, for example, officers suspect an individual, due to his or her erratic behavior, has been using drugs. In this case, the medical staff obtains and tests the sample with the on-site test kit, and, if found positive, the person can be more closely watched, or medical attention can be given more quickly.

> Small correctional facilities sometimes use on-site test kits for screening. With a test kit, facilities are able to get screening results immediately.

Biological Specimens

An additional practical consideration is the time frames that are inherent in testing different biological specimens. When hair is tested, the results of a one-and-one-half-inch hair sample typically indicate whether the tested individual has used a particular drug from a point in time starting about a week before the sample is taken to a point in time about three months earlier. Note that the hair sample has no information about drug use over the week before the sample was collected. The hair with that information is still below the surface of the scalp; it takes about a week for the growing hair to emerge to a point where the correctional staff person can cut it off. Hair has the longest drug-detection window (DDW) because it can give information about drug use from over the last several months. This result can be linked with the results of a urine test that typically measures drug use over the last one to three days and as recently as a couple of hours before the sample was collected.

What drug-test results can be expected if a parolee smoked crack in the parking lot just before submitting to a drug test but had not used the drug for ninety days before that? In the hair test, the cocaine would not have had time to show up. It is even possible that a urine test would be negative if the urine sample was collected within thirty minutes of the drug use. This is a largely theoretical point, however, because most parolees who smoke crack in the parking lot before coming for a drug test have also used it frequently in the days or weeks before the drug test. In that case, both the urine and hair drug-test results would be positive for cocaine.

Linking urine and hair tests together gives a more complete picture of the drug history of an individual than either test alone because of their different and complementary DDWs. There are significant advantages for correctional settings using multiple types of specimens to diagnose and monitor their offenders.

> There are significant advantages for correctional settings using multiple types of specimens to diagnose and monitor their offenders.

How Can a Medical Review Officer Help to Interpret Drug-Test Results?

Under some circumstances, the consequences of a positive laboratory test can be severe. For example, when an individual is court-ordered into treatment as a condition of his or her release, a series of positive laboratory-test results may mean that the judge will send the individual to jail. Because of this, a correctional facility might bring in a medical review officer, or MRO, to help interpret drug-test results. An MRO is a physician who is trained and certified to distinguish between drug abuse and medical use of similar or even identical substances. There is no need to gather a list of all medications that an individual is taking before collecting a sample for a drug test. Instead, a staff member of the program or an MRO needs only to investigate possible legitimate prescription use after getting a positive confirmatory test result. At that point, it is not necessary to ask about all the medicines the person may be using but only the specific drug or drugs identified from the drug test.

For example, suppose a young woman in her second year of college has been arrested on a DUI charge and released with a court order to have a drug and alcohol evaluation before sentencing. A urine sample could be taken at the evaluation center and sent to a commercial laboratory. Using the two-step testing approach, the result comes back positive for amphetamine. Rather than simply forwarding the test result to the courts, where the information can be used to prosecute her for taking illegal drugs, the evaluation center refers the case to an MRO. The MRO presents the result to the young woman, asking, very directly and simply, "Do you have a prescription for amphetamine?" noting that the most common reasons to take amphetamine medically are for narcolepsy, obesity, attention-deficit/hyperactivity disorder (ADHD), or as an adjunct to an antidepressant. If the college student professes to be under a physician's care for ADHD and has been prescribed Adderall, the MRO calls the prescribing physician to confirm the person's claim. Once that claim is verified by the prescribing physician, the MRO reports the drug-test result as negative. If the physician is unwilling to answer the MRO's question (a rare event even today), the person is asked to present the prescription bottle to the MRO. That bottle, by law, has on it the name of the person, the name of the prescribing physician, and the exact medicine that the physician prescribed for that person plus the date when the prescription was given to the person. Analogous to the use of confirming tests in drug testing, it is useful to have access to an MRO for complex or disputed drug-test results even though the MRO is seldom used.

> An MRO is a physician who is trained and certified to distinguish between drug abuse and medical use of similar or even identical substances.

How Accurate Is Drug Testing?

In the above example, it may seem as if both the screening and confirmatory tests were inaccurate. Actually, the results from the laboratory tests were perfectly accurate—there was amphetamine in the urine of the young woman. What needed to be determined was whether the amphetamine that was there was present by legal and legitimate means or from illegal use. The drug tests used today are 100 percent accurate in that they never identify a specimen that does *not* contain a drug as positive. In this case, the drugs were actually there—there was no inaccuracy in the drug identification. The MRO, in this case, helped to prevent a young woman from perhaps being more severely punished—or sent to a court-ordered treatment program for a drug she did not abuse.

This is an interesting example of a drug-testing problem that may confront a correctional setting. First, amphetamine is relatively seldom used as a street drug. When a person tests positive for recent use of a stimulant, it is usually cocaine or methamphetamine. Thus, testing positive for amphetamine should signal to corrections officers that there is something unusual about the case. Of course, if only a screening test were used, then the identification of amphetamine would not have been made. In the screening test, amphetamine and methamphetamine are linked as one single result. Only after a confirming test would the specific drug, amphetamine, be identified. Second, amphetamine most often, but not always, comes from a legitimate pharmaceutical manufacturer. It is a controlled substance; however, people can and do get addicted to it.

It's not uncommon for a college student to abuse prescription stimulants, especially amphetamine, and this college student may not be as innocent as she appears. Even if she has a prescription for amphetamine, she may be abusing it. Remember that the drug test does not reveal how much of the drug is present, only that it is present. An alert MRO will identify first whether the drug-test result reflects a legitimate prescription and, second, will explore with this person how the drug is being used.

> The drug test does not reveal how much of the drug is present, only that it is present.

As for the accuracy of drug tests in general, keep in mind that a person who uses a drug such as cocaine or marijuana infrequently or at low doses may produce a drug-test sample that is labeled negative for that drug. In such a case, either the drug was detected in the sample at a very low concentration that fell under the predetermined threshold, or cheating has occurred. The cutoff threshold is set at a relatively high level so that if a person has a concentration higher than that amount, there is no question that the tested person had been taking the drug and was not passively contaminated by it. The standard cutoff levels eliminate the "rock concert" excuse for marijuana positives: "I was at a rock concert, and people were smoking dope all around me!" As is the case with secondhand tobacco smoke, the person who is exposed to a drug someone else is smoking inhales it at levels too low to produce a positive drug-test result using current cutoff levels. One exception is infants who live in crack houses. They often test positive for cocaine, presumably because they are exposed to the drug environmentally and probably ingest fairly high concentrations because of contact with contaminated objects such as dishes and toys.

In disputed drug-test results, it is also possible that a mistake occurred in handling the specimen at the laboratory so that the test result reported for one individual is actually someone else's. A clerical error could have been made when a value was recorded or transmitted. These types of mistakes are rare, however, because laboratories have developed elaborate procedures to safeguard against them. Computers are used to follow samples through analysis, and results are often automatically recorded. Chain-of-custody procedures reduce the likelihood that a sample is mixed up between people because the security tags attached to the sample containers are signed and dated by the tested persons themselves.

When the laboratory takes samples to conduct specific tests, it takes the samples out of the individually labeled containers. The original signed containers are maintained even after all the testing is completed. If there is a reason to suspect that something went wrong somewhere and an incorrect result was reported, the original sample can be removed from the freezer, the signatures can be examined for authenticity, and another small amount can be removed from the container and retested at that same laboratory or even at a different laboratory.

> In disputed drug-test results, it is also possible that a mistake occurred in handling the specimen at the laboratory so that the test result reported for one individual is actually someone else's.

While errors are rare, they do occur, and it is wise to keep this possibility in mind when dealing with a disputed result. With respect to hair testing, it is possible to take a second sample within a week or two of the initial sample selection to confirm or refute the initial finding. It is not possible to do this with other samples—urine, oral fluids, or sweat patches—since the results are limited to specific times in the past. Hair is the exception because it grows slowly, and the evidence of recent drug use remains on the tested person's head for a few weeks.

> While errors are rare, they do occur, and it is wise to keep this possibility in mind when dealing with a disputed result.

Which Drugs Are Identified?

Drug-testing instruments are technically capable of detecting virtually any abused substance; however, only a few drugs are typically chosen as targets. This means that if a person sniffs glue or gasoline; takes GHB, LSD, or Ecstasy; or drinks lots of alcohol and the same day provides a urine sample for a typical drug test, he or she would get a negative result. This surprising outcome occurs because the typical drug test looks only for a small "test panel" of drugs. The test panel of the five most often-used drugs, called the SAMHSA-5, was derived over time by the Substance Abuse and Mental Health Services Administration (SAMHSA) to represent specific concerns and use in specific geographic areas. For example, phencyclidine (PCP) is rarely seen outside of Washington, D.C.; however, probably because PCP has been seen there, it is included in most drug-test panels administered nationwide. Other drugs on the typical test panel (originally developed for workplace testing) are based on more global concerns and include marijuana, cocaine, opiates (only morphine and codeine), and amphetamine/methamphetamine. Use of any other drug goes completely undetected.

Screening drug tests can be used for many other drugs, but because the preferred technology now is immunoassays, a specific antibody has to be developed to target that particular drug. If there is not much demand for the use of that particular drug antibody, then the cost per test is prohibitively high. The immunoassay antibodies are also proprietary so that the developer of a particular antibody for a specific drug can make it difficult for other companies to develop the same technology. Without competition, the cost of these drug tests remains high.

For the criminal justice system, this panel of five drugs is clearly inadequate. For offenders with a history of using other specific drugs—say synthetic opiates like OxyContin—it is essential that drugs such as these be tested for routinely. There is a smarter way to test for a wide range of drugs without incurring the cost of testing for many drugs on each sample. This approach has been used in the military for decades. It identifies the three drugs most often found and tests all samples for those three drugs. (A typical three-drug panel is marijuana, cocaine, and heroin, but in some places methamphetamine or PCP make the cut for the top three drugs.)

> These programs rotate the other drugs tested for with each sample so that the offenders being tested do not know which drugs they will be tested for when they give a sample.

These programs rotate the other drugs tested for with each sample so that the offenders being tested do not know which drugs they will be tested for when they give a sample. On this rotation list are drugs such as benzodiazepines, barbiturates, synthetic opiates, synthetic stimulants (such as methylphenidate), GHB, LSD, Ecstasy (MDMA), and any other drugs that are known to be used in the population being tested. With this rotation, depending on costs, two to four of these alternative drugs are included in the test battery for each sample. Over time, the program can easily identify emergent drugs of abuse and shift the frequency of testing to focus on those with the highest prevalence. It is desirable, however, to continue to include in a small percentage of the tests even drugs of low prevalence since drug-using patterns are subject to rapid changes over time, and only with regular (if infrequent) testing can a new drug be identified in the testing panel.

To disrupt cheating, it is desirable to use alternative samples instead of simply sticking with urine testing alone. When it comes to testing for a wide range of drugs, however, the preferred choice is urine since the alternative drug tests are still used on a relatively infrequent basis. That means that most test providers (laboratories and on-site test-kit manufacturers) focus solely on the basic five-drug panel. In the future, when testing other than urine testing becomes more common, a wider range of drugs will be able to be tested with the alternative specimens.

What to Test—Hair, Urine, Oral Fluids, or Sweat?

Hair

As mentioned earlier, hair has many advantages, including a very low likelihood of spreading disease. Hair samples are conveniently obtained, shipped, and stored because they do not require refrigeration. In addition, it is difficult to cheat or evade detection with hair tests, and hair tests produce semiquantitative results. Hair-sample collection is low in intrusiveness for the person. Hair uses the same two-step approach of drug testing, a screening test followed by a confirmatory GC/MS test, which is exactly the same as for all other drug-test specimen types.

When each bit of hair is formed in the hair follicle in the scalp, it incorporates the drugs that are in a person's blood. Head hair grows about one-half inch per month, and so a one-and-one-half-inch sample of hair measured from the scalp outward represents about ninety days of a DDW, or the amount of time covered by a drug test. If a person provided a hair sample that was three inches long, that would represent a DDW of six months. Since it takes about seven days for hair to emerge from the scalp, the DDW for hair does not include any drug use that took place in the seven days just prior to cutting the hair for a drug test. Cutting the hair is preferred because pulling the hair out by the roots is painful. A scissors is used to clip the hair as close to the scalp as possible. Hair strands are oriented in a collection container, and the ends nearest the head are identified. The laboratory then trims the excess hair off the specimen, retaining only the first one-and-one-half inches so that all routine hair samples reflect only the one-and-one-half inches of hair closest to the scalp. This standard has been adopted to level the playing field for tested subjects regardless of how long their hair is. The number of hairs retrieved for the test is about forty. People collecting hair

Hair has many advantages, including a very low likelihood of spreading disease.

samples do not count the hairs; rather, they twist some hair together high up at the back of the head until they have hairs about the thickness of a pencil lead. The cosmetic effect of sample collection on a person's hairstyle is so minor that it is difficult for anyone to identify the spot where the hair sample was taken. The results are expressed as positive or negative for each drug and represent any use during all of those last ninety days. It would be possible to divide the one-and-one-half-inch segment into three one-half-inch segments and then determine which months a person may have used a particular substance, but this is not usually done because the expense would triple the already-high cost of the hair test.

People who are bald or who have shaved their heads can have hair samples taken from their underarms, arms, legs, or back. Drugs are found in pubic hair, too, but this is seldom collected for obvious reasons. In cases where individuals have removed all other hair from their bodies, judges have ordered pubic hair collection. When hair other than head hair is used, there is less ability to link the positive result to a specific time frame, since hair other than head hair grows at a more unpredictable rate.

> **Unlike urine specimens, hair samples have more stable drug levels.**

Unlike urine specimens, hair samples have more stable drug levels. In fact, in one published study, a scientist working with the remains of a South American mummy discovered that the hair was positive for cocaine even though it had been thousands of years since that individual had last chewed coca leaves.

An important aspect of hair tests is that a "safety net" exists. If the person challenges the results, another sample can simply be taken. This is true because the hair segment last sampled is still there, waiting to be "harvested" again and again. Even if the person has shaved his or her head, the safety net can be used since body hair can be tested for drugs in this situation.

Hair tests do not detect a few isolated uses of a drug since the drug is not present in high-enough concentrations in the hair to be detected at the usual threshold. An individual must use a drug several times during that ninety-day DDW to produce a positive result. For marijuana, a person must use two or more times a week over the ninety-day DDW to be detected and labeled positive.

Finally, hair tests do not produce positive results for opiates after a person eats a poppy-seed bagel, as a urinalysis does. Poppy seeds naturally contain trace amounts of opiates; however, a hair-test specimen does not contain enough morphine or codeine to trigger a positive test result. On the other hand, it does not take many doses of heroin over ninety days to produce a positive result in a hair sample. The same is true for cocaine and methamphetamine.

Advantages of hair tests include the following:

- It's virtually impossible to cheat on the test.
- The DDW is long (usually ninety days).
- They permit discrimination between relatively limited and heavy use.
- Poppy-seed consumption does not give a positive drug-test result.
- Specimen collection is easy and poses no privacy issues.
- The specimens are not messy, unpleasant, or dangerous to handle or ship.
- In the case of disputed results, it's easy to retest within about two weeks of the initial test.

Disadvantages of hair tests include the following:

- They are more expensive than urine tests ($40 per test compared to $10).
- Fewer companies provide hair tests.
- There is no on-site drug-testing option (although some companies are currently attempting to develop this technology).
- The tests only detect repeated regular use of marijuana.

Urine

Urine testing dominates the drug-testing scene everywhere. Urine was the first type of specimen tested for drugs on a large scale. Because drugs are largely excreted through the kidneys and held in the bladder for elimination, the body concentrates drugs in the

Advantages of hair tests include the following:

- It's virtually impossible to cheat on the test.
- The DDW is long.
- Specimen collection is easy.
- In the case of disputed results, it's easy to retest.

urine, making it a logical sample for drug testing. Urine can be tested directly, so there is no need to prepare a sample for screening analysis, as is the case for hair and sweat testing.

Urine testing has a long history, with federal standards having been issued in 1988. These factors have made urine drug testing both more common and less controversial than other types of samples used for drug tests. The market itself has many suppliers of urine drug tests, and competition has driven prices down.

There are, however, some significant problems with urine tests. As mentioned earlier, the need for direct observation to prevent cheating has made this test relatively intrusive—the so-called "bathroom problem." Other strategies to avert cheating that do not involve direct observation are also problematic and easily circumvented. For example, test temperature strips that show how warm the liquid is inside the container can be circumvented by simply rubbing the test strip with a finger until the temperature is high enough—this allows a person to sneak in another person's urine and claim it as his or her own. Or a person being tested sometimes dilutes the sample with hot water from the faucet or even cold water from the toilet. Blue dye is sometimes added to the toilet water to prevent that water from being used, and the hot water is often just turned off to keep that water from being used.

> The need for direct observation to prevent cheating has made this test relatively intrusive—the so-called "bathroom problem."

An entire industry has emerged to help people cheat on urine tests. Test takers can add a product directly to the urine sample, confounding the test, or consume a pill purchased at a head shop before the test and supposedly disguise any drug present in the urine. The easiest way to beat the test, however, may still be the best—test subjects need only drink a large volume of water in the hours before the test. Water dilutes the concentration of any drugs present in the urine so that they fall below the cutoff levels. Although special laboratory tests have been created to compensate for this, they are not always used.

Because of the risk of cheating, some on-site tests now routinely identify creatinine, specific gravity, pH level, and three or four commonly used adulterants. Most commercial drug-testing laboratories offer these and other tests to detect cheating. We encourage correctional facilities to learn about cheating and to use drug tests, including special-order tests, wisely to detect and therefore discourage cheating. See chapter 6 for more information on cheating. Drug-testing laboratories and manufacturers of on-site test devices can help correctional facilities better recognize and deal with cheating.

Urine drug tests are usually reported as positive or negative without the semiquantitative results available for hair testing. With a urine test, a large amount of poppy seeds can trigger a positive drug-screen test for opiates. Since morphine and codeine are actually present in poppy seeds in very small quantities, chemists do not consider the result a false positive.

Poppy seeds confounding the drug test for opiates can be a problem in a community corrections setting, but it is seldom, if ever, a significant problem in incarceration situations, where offenders can be prevented from eating large amounts of poppy seeds. In community corrections settings, it is important that the laboratory or the on-site tests use the 300-nanogram cutoff for morphine and codeine and not the 2,000-nanogram cutoff that is now used in workplace drug testing. Using the higher cutoffs causes many otherwise positive urine tests produced by recent heroin users to be missed.

Advantages of urine tests include the following:

- Urine is the most widely used sample for drug testing; therefore, urine testing has the largest body of experience and has been subject to the most extensive legal review.

- Urine is the least expensive sample to use; the per-test cost is the lowest of any samples.

- When using urine testing, the correctional facility has the largest number of potential suppliers of tests for on-site and laboratory drug testing.

- For those wanting to test beyond the SAMHSA-5 drug panel, urine offers the largest range of options for drug identification.

Advantages of urine tests include the following:

- Urine is the most widely used sample for drug testing.
- Urine is the least expensive sample to use.
- Urine offers the largest range of options for drug identification.

Disadvantages of urine tests include the following:

- Urine is the sample that is most easy to cheat with.
- Urine has a short DDW, usually one to three days after drug use, although some urine drug tests are negative twelve hours after the last drug use.
- Poppy seeds can produce the same positive result as heroin, so not only would a false positive be produced if heroin were not being used, but heroin use would not be identified if poppy seeds had been consumed recently.
- Urine collection is comparatively intrusive.
- Urine is messy, unpleasant, and (given its potential to harbor pathogens) dangerous to handle, ship, and store.
- It is impossible to obtain another specimen of urine for the same time period.

Oral Fluids

Drug testing with oral fluids is a newer technique. A swab or piece of absorbent material is placed in the person's mouth for about a minute and then placed in a collection container. If an on-site test is done, the patch is squeezed mechanically and the fluid from the mouth is forced into a chamber, where it reacts with specific drug-detection antibodies. The results can be read in a few minutes. If the test is positive, the entire vessel can be shipped to a laboratory for confirmation testing. The initial oral-fluids test can, of course, also be done at a laboratory and not on-site.

> Drug testing with oral fluids is a newer technique.

Because oral fluids, including saliva, are in equilibrium or in balance with the blood, they are effective in identifying recent use of the commonly studied drugs. The exception is for marijuana, since the available on-site oral-fluids testing kits lack the sensitivity of the laboratory testing of oral fluids. However, put into perspective, no drug test will identify everyone who has recently consumed marijuana or any other drug of abuse.

Advantages of oral-fluids testing include the following:

- It provides easy collection.
- It poses no privacy issues.

- The tests are resistant to cheating.
- On-site options are available.
- The cost is comparable to urine tests (less than hair tests).

Disadvantages of oral-fluids testing include the following:

- It is not sensitive to marijuana, especially in on-site tests.
- There is less experience with it than with urine or hair tests.
- It has a short DDW (twelve to twenty-four hours).

Sweat Patch

Sweat-patch testing is less often used in correctional settings since it does little to help identify past exposure to drugs. The patch can only identify current drug use. It can be used to monitor drug use while a person is in court-ordered drug-abuse treatment or in a parole/probation setting. The patch is worn for one or two weeks at a time. As a person sweats, the patch picks up any traces of drugs that leave the bloodstream and exit the pores with perspiration. The water in sweat evaporates through the membrane on the outside of the patch, but the traces of drugs are caught inside the patch, where they are retained. The patch is removed from the person's skin and sent to a laboratory for testing. The drugs in the patch are dissolved and analyzed for the presence of specific drugs using the same immunoassay screen and GC/MS confirmation technology that is used for all other drug tests.

The sweat patch is highly resistant to cheating because if the person tampers with the patch, the edges pucker in ways that cannot be disguised. The patch cannot be temporarily removed without destroying the safety seal, preventing people from taking the patch off for a time to use drugs. Tampering may not mean that a person has actually used any drugs, only that he or she may have considered removing it for that reason.

Advantages of sweat-patch testing include the following:

- It provides easy collection.
- It poses no privacy issues.
- The tests are resistant to cheating.

> The sweat patch is highly resistant to cheating because if the person tampers with the patch, the edges pucker in ways that cannot be disguised.

- The cost is comparable to urine tests (less than hair tests).
- It has a long DDW (up to several weeks, depending on how long the patch is worn).
- Sweat-patch tests look forward from the time the patch is put on, not backward from collection as do all other drug tests.

Disadvantages of sweat-patch testing include the following:

- It collects information on drug use only after the patch is applied.
- There is less experience with it than with urine or hair tests.
- The patch is painful to remove when placed over body hairs.

Which Drug Tests Are the Best?

No one test is clearly better in all applications. Our recommendation to any correctional setting is that it use all four of the major specimens: urine, hair, sweat, and oral fluids. The overall system and the underlying science of drug testing are sound. Each of the commonly used samples has its strengths and weaknesses. Urine tests are the least expensive, the most widely used, and the easiest for which to find on-site or laboratory providers, often ones that are local to the correctional setting. These are real advantages that explain why correctional settings do more urine testing than any other form of drug tests. However, urine testing gets drug testing into the bathroom, it is relatively easy to cheat on, and it cannot separate heroin use from poppy-seed consumption.

Hair testing is becoming more widely used because it has a long DDW (ninety days), the samples are easily collected without going into a bathroom, and the tests are virtually impossible to cheat on. Hair testing is more expensive on a per-test basis. However, when considered with respect to the amount of information obtained from that one test, the cost-benefit ratio (discussed later in this chapter) changes significantly in favor of hair tests.

Oral-fluids testing is also being adopted in more correctional settings because it does not have the bathroom-privacy problem, it is resistant to cheating, it is relatively affordable, and it can be done

> No one test is clearly better in all applications. Our recommendation to any correctional setting is that it use all four of the major specimens: urine, hair, sweat, and oral fluids.

on-site. However, oral fluids are relatively insensitive to marijuana and have a short DDW (twelve to twenty-four hours).

Sweat patches are increasingly being used in correctional settings for monitoring offenders' drug use while they are on parole/probation. Since the patch cannot detect drug use before it is applied, it cannot be used in assessment of past use during criminal-intake protocols.

Sweat patches are increasingly being used in correctional settings for monitoring offenders' drug use while they are on parole/probation.

We recommend that correctional settings use a combination of all of these drug tests and tailor testing to meet the needs of the correctional setting and the offender. For example: On-site testing of oral fluids might work best in monitoring compliance in a parole or probation program, whereas hair testing might work best when diagnosing the long-term drug history of a person coming into a court-ordered treatment program and when confirming abstinence over a long period of time in a population of offenders with low risk of drug use, such as people nearing the end of a court-ordered treatment program.

Sweat patches might be used to monitor drug use in a parole or probation program when parole officers suspect that a person is simply abstaining from use in the days before a scheduled appointment when a urine test will be given. Urine tests might be the best alternative when individuals are not able to provide a hair sample from their heads and you are able to conduct frequent random tests in a carefully controlled environment such as a prison setting. Urine may also be the best choice when relatively unusual drugs are being detected, since it is easier to get special-order urine tests.

Improving the Cost-Benefit Performance of Drug Testing

Within the criminal justice setting, there are several reasons for conducting drug tests. The primary one is to learn the truth about an offender's drug use. In this way, corrections staff can arrange for services to be provided to that individual, reducing the chance he or she will recidivate. Staff members cannot find out the exact dimensions of a person's problem simply by asking.

Typically, during the pretrial stage, it is important to know how much and what types of drugs an offender might have used over the last few months. Using a drug test to look back over the past three months would be very useful since it would identify a pattern of behavior. It would also be important to be able to distinguish between experimental and heavy use. Such a drug test would have maximum information value since the amount of information derived from one drug test could be used to create a comprehensive substance-abuse summary for use in court.

One way to scale this information benefit is simply to multiply a drug test's DDW by the relative benefit of having quantitative, semiquantitative, or qualitative information for each of the drugs of interest. This will reveal something about the informational benefit associated with that particular drug test.

Application: Long-Term Historical Use Indicator

To begin this discussion of cost-benefit ratios, we will focus first on the long-term historical use that might be the basis of a pretrial diagnostic test. Then we will expand the discussion to include a recalculation of the cost-benefit ratios when considering the two other most common applications: monitoring and immediate.

Dividing the cost of doing a drug test by the quantified informational benefits gives us the cost-benefit ratio that we can use to compare all drug tests. Note, however, that in this analysis, preference is given to drug tests that have the ability to give us the longest historical drug-use information (their DDW). This might not always be the most important consideration depending on how the test information will be used—for example, if results must be learned immediately.

To begin this first example, we will explicitly calculate the cost-benefit ratio for urine drug tests when used as a long-term historical use indicator. First, we note our cost: we can obtain the standard five-drug panel of tests with confirmation of all positives for $10 when our agency establishes a contract with a local urinalysis laboratory. Second, we calculate the benefit of such a test when attempting to assess long-term historical use by using the following

> Dividing the cost of doing a drug test by the quantified informational benefits gives us the cost-benefit ratio that we can use to compare all drug tests.

formula: DDW x result code x the number of drugs in panel = informational benefit. Note that the result code is either qualitative (coded as 1), semiquantitative (coded as 2), or quantitative (coded as 3). In this case, each drug that we are testing for can be detected for 2 days, and the result is multiplied by the qualitative test result of 1. So 2 x 1 = 2 for each drug, multiplied by the 5 drugs in the panel, gives us a quantified informational benefit of (2 x 5 =) 10.

Finally, in step three, we calculate the ratio by simply dividing the cost ($10) by the benefits (10) to get a cost-benefit ratio of (10 ÷ 10 =) 1.00. To interpret this, we could say that urine tests have a cost-benefit ratio of $1.00 per informational benefit. Table 3 below summarizes the cost-benefit ratios of several types of drug tests for different uses.

TABLE 3

Cost-to-Informational-Benefit Ratios			
Type of Drug Test	Long-Term Historical Use Application	Monitoring Application	Immediate Application
Urine	1.00	0.50	N/A
Hair	0.07*	0.05*	N/A
Oral Fluids	0.92	0.46	0.92*
Sweat	N/A	0.10	N/A

* Indicates lowest cost per informational benefit

We can interpret this tabled information as follows: given that we are interested in using a drug test to assess long-term historical drug use, the most expensive cost per benefit is the urine drug test, with a score of 1.00. A drug test that is somewhat better is the oral-fluids test, with a score of 0.92, and the best drug test in the cost-benefit analysis is the hair test, with a score of 0.07. Note that the sweat-patch test is not applicable in the long-term historical use indicator category since it measures drug use prospectively, not retrospectively, as would be required when doing a diagnostic test on a pretrial inmate.

Application: Monitoring Indicator

When calculating the cost-benefit ratio for the next major application, condition of monitoring, we are concerned about the drug use of an individual while he or she is under drug-court supervision or on probation or parole. Here we would also be interested in detecting a relapse condition in order to appropriately respond. Within this type of application, criminal justice agencies most often use a randomized drug-testing procedure where not everyone gets tested every week. Since offenders never know exactly when they will be tested, they are motivated to stay clean just in case they may be tested. This psychological manipulation generally works very well and can dramatically reduce the overall drug-testing costs associated with monitoring. So instead of routine weekly urine or oral-fluids tests for all offenders, a program can effectively monitor and motivate people with a random twice-monthly regimen.

Using the same formula as on page 59, with an adjustment for the psychological impact of the random-testing schedule as equivalent to four tests per month, we divide the total cost for the month ($20.00) by the benefits (40) and get a cost-benefit ratio for urine in the monitoring application environment of 0.50. The results of this analysis in the monitoring application are also shown in table 3. Note that the cost-benefit ratio of hair is the best with a cost-to-informational-benefit score of 0.05, with sweat patches close behind at 0.10. Oral fluids had the next-highest cost per benefit with 0.46, and urine was the highest (most expensive) with a score of 0.50. Sweat patches can be worn for up to two weeks, so two patches would be needed to monitor someone for one month. (We are assuming that a patch is placed on a person at the beginning of the month of interest and then changed and examined midmonth.) This gives the psychological equivalent benefit of a routine or weekly monitoring program.

> Since offenders never know exactly when they will be tested, they are motivated to stay clean just in case they may be tested.

Hair tests would only be done once per month to cover every day in that month and would be seen to offer the same psychological motivation to stay clean as a routine weekly testing program.

Application: Immediate Indicator

Finally, the cost-benefit ratios can be calculated for the immediate criminal justice system need. In this scenario, the agency must have an immediate answer as to whether the person involved is currently under the influence of some drug. This would be necessary when an offender presents himself or herself at a probation, parole, or drug-court facility and appears to be intoxicated. This situation has a need for immediacy for several reasons. First, the offender may not be able to drive safely and may need to be taken home. Second, the offender may have to be arrested for violation of court-ordered drug abstinence and taken to jail to await a judge's decision. Perhaps because of other prescription medications or medical conditions, the offender may need immediate medical attention. There may also be other reasons why probation/parole officers need to have an immediate answer as to whether a person is intoxicated. These for-cause testing applications within criminal justice agencies are critical since they allow law enforcement to immediately take the correct steps to ensure that appropriate actions are taken.

Calculating the cost-benefit ratio in the immediate application is limited only to oral fluids because drugs are not available in hair, urine, or sweat quickly enough for detection. For example, when an offender smoked crack in the parking lot just before presenting himself to his probation officer, the officer noticed that he was acting strangely and asked him to take an oral-fluids test. Since inhaled cocaine vapors are nearly immediately available to the blood plasma of that individual, cocaine can be detected in his oral fluids within two minutes of drug use. Had a urine test been ordered, the drug would not be present in detectable amounts in the urine for at least twenty minutes, and the test would be negative. Hair testing would not be appropriate here at all since it would take seven days for the drug to be incorporated into the hair matrix and then grow out of

Calculating the cost-benefit ratio in the immediate application is limited only to oral fluids because drugs are not available in hair, urine, or sweat quickly enough for detection.

the scalp far enough to be recovered by scissors. So in table 3 (see page 59) we see that none of the drug-test types are applicable for this application with the exception of oral fluids.

The oral-fluids cost-benefit ratio here is calculated as the cost of $11 for a 6-drug panel, divided by the DDW of 2 days, multiplied by the qualitative result multiplier of 1 for each of the 6 drugs in the panel: $11 \div ([2 \times 1] 6) = 0.92$. Considering that this is the only type of test that can respond to this unique situation of crack cocaine use in the parking lot just prior to an appointment with a probation officer, the cost-benefit ratio is probably not important. Rather, this table demonstrates clearly that each of these types of tests is probably useful in a particular setting because of its inherent strengths and not useful in other settings because of its inherent weaknesses.

In Summary: Costs to Informational Benefits

In general, hair testing appears to have the most informational benefits per dollar when the criminal justice agency is concerned with obtaining long-term historical information on drug use during a diagnostic test of pretrial inmates. It also appears to have the most informational benefits per dollar when the agency is concerned with monitoring drug use during the time an offender is in a community release program or is incarcerated. However, when an immediate need exists to determine whether an individual is actively intoxicated with drugs, only oral-fluids testing can provide an answer.

No one type of drug test is the best at doing everything.

The most important lesson from this discussion of cost-to-informational-benefit ratios for each type of test is that every criminal justice agency will need to utilize many different types for each of a number of different applications. No one type of drug test is the best at doing everything; providing the best information for adjudication will mean utilizing the most appropriate tool at the appropriate time. Decisions can also be made to lower drug-testing costs by converting a testing program to another type of test, using table 3 to select an alternate test that still provides an informational benefit that comes closest to the ideal.

Other Improvements to the Cost-Benefit Performance

A simple way to lower costs associated with a drug-testing program is to maximize admission of drug use as an alternative to testing. For example, when an offender presents himself at his probation office, the officer can hold the urine cup or scissors in his hand and ask, "Have you been using? How much? How often?" and then tell the probationer, "You might as well just tell me [looking at collection cup]. I'll find out with this, and you can save us both some time by just admitting what is going on." If the probation officer has established a good rapport with the offender, the admission of some use may be close to the results of the bioassay. Naturally, a probation officer could not do this every time, since the offender will simply begin to lie without any fear of eventually being discovered. But this technique may allow an agency to reduce its overall testing costs by about a third, while continuing to learn about most offenders' drug use.

Another obvious way to begin to control costs is to create an administrative monitoring system that records all results and costs. In this way, it might be discovered that a particular drug that was always tested for had only two positives (out of several thousand tests) in the previous year. It becomes an easy decision, then, to drop that one drug from the urinalysis panel and save about one-fifth of the total bioassay costs.

Finally, another proven way to reduce an agency's direct costs of operating a drug-testing program is to justify those costs as part of various grant applications and let the funding agency bear the costs for the duration of the new project. For example, when a local sheriff wanted an epidemiological study of drug use conducted as part of the booking process in the jail that he operated, it was possible to obtain federal grant money that covered this cost as part of a research project on drug-detection technologies.

> A simple way to lower costs associated with a drug-testing program is to maximize admission of drug use as an alternative to testing.

5

. . . . .

Managing a Drug-Testing Program
in Correctional Settings

In this chapter, we'll look at the practical aspects of managing a drug-testing program in a correctional setting. No one method works best in all correctional settings, but certain considerations are important in all drug-testing operations. One goal of court-ordered drug-abuse treatment is abstinence from the use of alcohol and other drugs. For many people, abstinence is unlikely to be sustained without drug testing, which can be a means of accountability and reinforcement.

Drug testing must be built into all aspects of the criminal justice system. On any given day, about four million people in the community are under the supervision of the criminal justice system. More than half of them regularly use illegal drugs. This makes drug testing critical. But to be successful, drug testing needs the active support of the management at each criminal justice agency.

Identifying a Drug-Testing Coordinator

To ensure that each criminal justice facility has a good drug-testing program, we encourage the identification of one person to function as the drug-testing coordinator (DTC) for that agency. This staff member should be responsible for understanding how drug testing works, for knowing which of the many testing options are available to the program, and for the day-to-day management of drug-testing operations. The DTC can work with other correctional programs to learn how they use drug testing and to compare best practices. In addition, the DTC can establish positive working alliances with local drug-testing programs, including those used by major employers as well as drug-abuse treatment programs and schools. Other drug-testing sites—both locally and nationally—can also be useful to the drug-testing program in many ways, including helping to find the best tests and the best deals on drug tests. Finally, we encourage the DTC to evaluate the drug-testing program and to report the major findings to the public. Not only will evaluation and research help to improve the effectiveness of the correctional program, but drug-testing results will also be valuable to public health and law-enforcement efforts in the wider community. For a summary of the roles of the DTC, see table 4 below.

> The DTC can establish positive working alliances with local drug-testing programs.

TABLE 4

The Roles of the Drug-Testing Coordinator in a Criminal Justice System Agency
1. Oversee the drug-testing program for the agency
2. Select and advise in the purchasing of the drug tests to be used in the agency
3. Keep up-to-date with the evolving technology of drug testing and provide training to others in the agency
4. Record and report the results of the drug tests for the agency as a whole for outcome reporting as well as forecasting
5. Answer questions about drug tests for leadership, staff, prisoners, offenders, detainees, and the public
6. Keep in touch with other people using drug tests to stay current and to find the best products at the best prices
7. Network with other drug-testing providers

We recognize that most criminal justice agencies may not be able to afford a full-time position devoted to drug testing. Therefore, we suggest that the agency leadership pick a widely respected, hard-working, and well-motivated staff member to add this role to his or her other duties. Having a single person, even in a part-time role, who is charged with this responsibility is important, because without this designation it is too easy for everyone (and therefore for no one) to take the responsibility for managing the drug testing in the criminal justice agency. Having one person with this responsibility also makes it possible for that person to do the work needed to learn about drug testing and how best to do it. The DTC can interact with the laboratories and drug-test suppliers that the agency uses, as well as with other organizations in the community using drug testing.

How to Test

Within correctional settings, there are two distinct types of drug testing: *random testing* and *for-cause testing*. Random testing occurs on a predetermined schedule established by the correctional facility, with the frequency of the random testing being based on the expectation that a particular offender, or a population of offenders, is likely to use drugs. The more likely the drug use, the more frequent the random testing. For this reason, random testing is more frequent during the initial stages of working with an offender and less frequent after months of stable abstinence. As long as a person is in a court-ordered drug-abuse treatment program, it is desirable to continue random drug testing, even if the frequency of that testing is low late in recovery.

> Within correctional settings, there are two distinct types of drug testing: *random testing* and *for-cause testing*.

In addition to random testing, which occurs on a schedule determined by a software program so as to be truly random, for-cause testing occurs whenever anyone on the corrections program staff has reason to suspect a particular person may have recently used alcohol or other drugs. Examples of triggers for for-cause drug testing are offenders missing probation meetings or appearing intoxicated or hungover. It is important that all drug tests be labeled either random or for-cause so that the results of these two forms of tests are separated during evaluation. In general, the likelihood of a for-cause test being positive is high, often as much as 50 percent or more. In contrast, most random tests are negative, often 5 percent to 10 percent positive. The random tests give the corrections facility a better idea of the level of drug use in the offender population, with the frequency of positive tests being inversely proportional to the duration of court-ordered treatment, meaning the offenders who have been in treatment the longest have the lowest average rate of positive drug-test results. Frequent drug testing raises the offenders' odds of success in drug-abuse treatment.

As a starting point in establishing or reviewing a drug-testing operation, the corrections facility staff or the DTC needs to decide which drug tests to use under which circumstances. For example, the DTC must determine if the program has the necessary equipment and utilities to use certain tests. Having access to restrooms is important for urine testing. Some correctional agencies share a building, and its restrooms, with other tenants, who may be upset that people are frequenting the bathroom and that staff members sometimes have to observe urinating offenders. If there are messes in or vandalism to the bathroom, the correctional agency is most likely the first to be blamed. When considering urine testing, try, if at all possible, to have the restrooms on-site.

When choosing urine testing as the primary method of drug testing, you need to consider whether to observe the process directly to prevent cheating. The single best way to reduce cheating on urine drug tests is to carefully, closely, and directly observe the urine going from the donor into the collection cup. Direct observation eliminates most of the major cheating strategies. If you suspect that the donor of a urine sample has cheated, there are three good options to consider at the time of collection: (1) repeat the sample collection under careful, direct supervision, (2) immediately collect an oral-fluids sample, or (3) conduct a hair test. Either of the first two approaches cover the time immediately before the test, while the hair test covers the previous ninety days minus the seven days just prior to the test.

> As a starting point in establishing or reviewing a drug-testing operation, the corrections facility staff or the DTC needs to decide which drug tests to use under which circumstances.

If cheating is thought to be covering up only very recent use, the hair-test option is not appropriate.

Observations can be uncomfortable for all parties involved. Positioning mirrors so that the observer does not have to look directly at the person but still can see him or her urinate in the bottle can reduce some discomfort. Mirrors are helpful if the restroom is small or if the person is in a stall and there is not enough room for two people. Other possibilities are video cameras or one-way mirrors from adjacent rooms. These are options, but sometimes they are cost prohibitive, and they can be abused by those who are not authorized to use the equipment or be in the observation room.

Managing how the drug-testing procedure is implemented can reduce confusion and mistakes. This is critical when test results have serious consequences, such as a prison sentence. A person in a court-ordered drug-treatment program may find himself or herself in custody as a result of a positive test because of the mishandling of samples or errors of recording results. It is important to have standard procedures that are followed at all times. The National Institute on Drug Abuse (NIDA) has developed a chain-of-custody form that suggests a procedure that can be followed from the time the urine-analysis (UA) bottle leaves the technician's hand to when it is sent to be tested by a laboratory. For example, a bottle is given to an offender for a urine sample. The offender is asked to empty his or her pockets and leave jackets, bags, or purses outside the restroom. This obviously would not be a significant issue in a prison setting. Trays are available to put items on so they do not get lost or misplaced.

> Managing how the drug-testing procedure is implemented can reduce confusion and mistakes. This is critical when test results have serious consequences, such as a prison sentence.

After collection, the offender returns with the sample and hands it to the technician. Labels are either printed up from computer software that tracks the sample or are handwritten by the technician. The name of the offender, the date, the time it was collected, and the signatures of the technician and the offender are on the label. Once the sample is given to the person collecting it, it is not set in a box or on a shelf to be labeled at another time, but is labeled immediately, in the presence of the offender. This prevents the bottle from getting mixed up with someone else's, and because the offender observes the labeling process, he or she can validate its accuracy. The lid is checked to make sure it is secure; leaving a loose cap on the bottle is often done intentionally by offenders seeking to foil the test. The hope is that, by the time the bottle reaches the testing site, most of the urine will have spilled out. Any time urine samples are handled, the technicians receiving the bottles should wear rubber gloves to protect themselves from hepatitis and other easily transmitted diseases.

The technician wraps a security strip over the cap and places the label around the bottle and security strip. At that time, the offender initials the security strip and the collector signs the label. This procedure ensures that the sample came from the offender and that it will not be tampered with by anyone until it reaches the lab to be processed. It also minimizes claims that someone mixed up the bottles or put something in the sample to make it positive.

The sample is placed in a plastic bag and sealed. It is then dropped in a secured container to which offenders have no access. This could be a locked cabinet or a box on a shelf in a room to which only staff has access. For off-site testing, all the samples are bagged in a larger container just prior to pickup by a courier. A list of all the names on the samples is placed in the bag and sealed. Once again, what is in the bag and on the list prevents tampering or confusion. This procedure is the same for any other drug test that has to be collected and sent to a laboratory, including those using hair and oral-fluids samples.

A streamlined system, preferably a database where information is stored and easily accessed by authorized personnel, is most helpful for recording who is being tested and how often. This information is useful when correctional facilities are preparing outcome and evaluation reports. An administrative assistant or the DTC can input this information into the database daily or weekly. Often, drug-testing laboratories provide the software needed to print container labels and to keep track of results. The laboratory can also set up online accounts to receive drug-test results. This cuts down on delays resulting from mailing or faxing the information.

> A streamlined system, preferably a database where information is stored and easily accessed by authorized personnel, is most helpful for recording who is being tested and how often.

The importance of establishing a timely and efficient procedure to notify corrections staff of test results should not be underestimated. First, the DTC records the test results in the offender's records. The DTC then notifies corrections staff regarding the status of the offender's drug use. Efficiency and timing are crucial. Receiving reports one to three weeks after sample collection is frustrating for the corrections staff and may slow down the legal process. The sooner a corrections staff member has information that an offender tested positive, the greater the likelihood of intervening before a full-blown relapse or before the person can commit other drug-related crimes.

> The importance of establishing a timely and efficient procedure to notify corrections staff of test results should not be underestimated.

Whom to Test

Drug testing in the criminal justice population has far fewer complications than drug testing in most other situations. For example, upon court order, an offender can be compelled to provide a urine sample, provide a hair sample, provide an oral-fluids sample, and wear a sweat patch. There have been instances where offenders have shaved their head hair to avoid a court-ordered hair test only to be removed from the courtroom so a bailiff can cut their pubic hair for testing. Such requirements for compliance and sanctions that include jail time for noncompliance simply don't exist in other settings such as drug-treatment programs, schools, and the workplace. Because there are few limitations in the criminal justice system on who is eligible to be tested, and since offenders must comply or face serious sanctions, the issue is who should be tested based on cost-effectiveness.

Pretrial offenders are typically tested to establish their pattern of drug use at the time of and just prior to their arrest. This is both a diagnostic as well as forensic test, since the results will be used in both ways. For example, as a diagnostic test, drug tests provide the courts information critical to making disposition decisions, including referral to other services and diversion programs as alternatives to incarceration. The results of these drug tests are critical to properly placing individuals into the correct program or facility. As such, all pretrial offenders could be tested with results sent to the court. However, testing all individuals who are in the pretrial stage is expensive.

One way to control costs of the drug-testing program among the pretrial population would be to limit court-ordered testing to offenders with certain charges that might benefit from court-ordered services implemented postconviction. This would include all offenders brought up on nonviolent felony charges and all cases involving drug possession. Persons facing these charges and those individuals who are known to be involved with drugs (including those with alcohol violations and DUIs) should be given these tests so that they might be included in in-jail or in-prison treatment programs as well as possible diversion to other outside treatment programs with attendance as a condition for release. (According to these limitations, people with violent charges should not be tested since they are unlikely to be released into outside drug-treatment agencies and are unlikely to be eligible to participate in in-jail or in-prison treatment programs or receive other treatment services.) However, if the forensic applications of the drug tests are being considered, those individuals who have violent crime charges that involve drug use as a contributing element should be tested so that the court can consider adjusting their sentences accordingly.

The one group of pretrial offenders that would not have to be drug tested would be misdemeanants who do not have any drug possession or alcohol violation charges. This decision is made only on the cost-effectiveness of operating the drug-testing program and not on the potential benefits that some few misdemeanants may see as a result of all individuals being tested. For example, someone arrested for loitering may be involved with drugs and might benefit from court-ordered drug testing, since it would mean that individual could be ordered into treatment. However, testing such individuals could make the total drug-testing program costs prohibitively expensive.

Among the offenders who have been convicted of any felony or any drug charge, a monitoring program of drug tests should be

> One way to control costs of the drug-testing program among the pretrial population would be to limit court-ordered testing to offenders with certain charges that might benefit from court-ordered services implemented postconviction.

initiated if their pretrial drug test showed that they were positive for at least one illegal drug—or if they admitted to drug use during the court proceedings. If convicted felons did not test positive for any drugs during their pretrial diagnostic or forensic evaluations, then to maximize the cost-effectiveness of the program, these individuals would not have to be tested as part of a routine drug-test monitoring program.

Finally, all individuals who are in community release programs such as probation, parole, and drug-court supervision should be randomly drug tested on a regular basis with all results evaluated by the courts or probation and parole officers to decide whether to terminate participation in the program and begin incarceration. Some of these offenders will test positive as they work through their recovery, and therefore it should be left up to the discretion of the professionals whether to send the offender back to jail based on their assessment of whether that offender is making satisfactory progress. Because relapse is often a part of recovery, a single positive test is often not considered enough reason to send an offender to jail.

A special note regarding juvenile offenders: drug testing minors should be done under the same circumstances as has been described for adults. As pretrial detainees, juveniles are currently offered a drug test in some jurisdictions, and compliance is strictly voluntary. Some juvenile justice agencies claim to have a very high rate of cooperation in getting juveniles to participate in a drug test even when they know that the results will be used by the courts to refer them to drug treatment.

> Drug testing minors should be done under the same circumstances as has been described for adults.

What Test to Use

In retrospect, it is obvious that when Elizabeth (see chapter 3) came into the jail's booking area and began acting out, a voluntary drug test administered as soon as possible by the medical evaluation staff could have prevented her death. The issue of what test to use becomes important when considering the defining characteristics of the situation and the reason for conducting the test. Elizabeth showed every symptom of intoxication: she was physically unstable, incoherent, combative, and argumentative; she was speaking too loudly and had the odor of alcohol about her. In such a medically urgent situation, the drug test should be conducted in a way that will give medical staff immediate information, ensuring that the offender receives appropriate treatment. A urine test could have been done, but given that Elizabeth was combative and argumentative, it is unlikely that she would have complied with a request to urinate into a collection cup in the ladies' room. A hair test could have been taken, but the sample would have to be sent to a laboratory, and the results would not have been known for several days. Likewise, a sweat patch would be inappropriate, since it collects information on drug use prospectively rather than retrospectively. Therefore, the best alternative was to take an oral-fluids sample and analyze the sample immediately with an on-site test kit. The discovery of cocaine and heroin in her saliva would have then initiated a very different handling protocol, whereby she would have been put under intense observation by both medical and correctional staff and eventually, as the effects of the drugs she had taken became more pronounced, she would have been sent to the local hospital. This would have saved Elizabeth's life.

In other cases, the pretrial population might be better served by taking urine samples and having the specimens analyzed at a local laboratory, where results can be available to the courts within two days. In cases where the justification for the test is forensic (for example, violent crimes), court-ordered hair specimens would provide better and more complete information about an individual's pattern of drug use during the last ninety days. This would be especially important to the court if the crime had been committed during that time frame, since drug use might then be argued to be a contributing factor. Using hair to drug test all people with nonviolent charges and no drug offenses while they are in the pretrial stage would be prohibitively expensive, even though there is a possibility that many drug users in that group would benefit from identification and

> In cases where the justification for the test is forensic, court-ordered hair specimens would provide better and more complete information about an individual's pattern of drug use during the last ninety days.

subsequent treatment. While we would like to advocate that everyone involved in the criminal justice system be court-ordered for drug testing on entry, we realize that hard choices must be made when limited funds are available to administer such a program. What we have suggested, therefore, is a reality-based compromise between the ideal and what we consider to be the absolute minimum.

For offenders who are under court supervision, this drug-testing program would be administered in a monitoring capacity. Here the choice of what test to use can be modified to suit each offender's situation. For example, if an offender is in prison or in jail, a random test program using frequent urinalysis would be effective at discouraging institutional drug use. Using hair tests would also be an effective way to monitor drug use in the institution, since it would only have to be done infrequently to cover a long period of time. This would mean cutting a hair sample from the individual's head every month or perhaps every two or three months. Since these individuals are incarcerated, it would also be possible to effectively implement a sweat-patch-based drug-testing program. In this instance, offenders would be required to wear the patch for one or two weeks, then it would be removed and tested either on-site or sent to a laboratory for analysis. Oral fluids should probably not be used as part of a drug-monitoring program since they only detect drugs that have been used over the last day or so, and even if these tests are administered as part of a random selection process, the costs to achieve the same level of coverage provided by other methods would be prohibitive. Oral-fluids tests should be on hand, however, to be used when correction officers or guards see behavior that makes them suspect that a particular inmate has recently used drugs.

For individuals in postconviction community release programs, which include probation, parole, and drug-court supervision, the type of drug test that should be used depends on the degree of expected compliance. That is, when an offender first reports to a probation officer and is court mandated to be tested, the probation officer should select a test that will not only provide information over all

> For offenders who are under court supervision, this drug-testing program would be administered in a monitoring capacity. Here the choice of what test to use can be modified to suit each offender's situation.

or most of the time before his or her next appointment, but also will inexpensively match this information to that time frame. Two good ways to conduct this community-based drug monitoring are with a sweat patch or a hair test. The sweat patch would be useful if the offender is to be seen initially every one or two weeks. If the expected time between meetings is one month or more, then only the hair test can cover that length of time without more frequent contact.

The types of drugs that an agency might test for include the standard marijuana, cocaine, morphine/codeine, amphetamine/methamphetamine, and phencyclidine (PCP). As mentioned earlier, because this list was developed in the mid-1980s, it does not include drugs that have since become very popular. A list of commonly used drugs that are not in this standard panel contains dozens of other drugs. One way to decide which drugs to test for on a routine basis within any jurisdiction is to conduct an epidemiological study covering a wide range of substances. Offenders could also be interviewed as well as narcotics officers. This information could then be used to develop a list of drugs of concern that are unique to that particular jurisdiction.

> One way to decide which drugs to test for on a routine basis within any jurisdiction is to conduct an epidemiological study covering a wide range of substances.

When to Test

How often a drug test is administered is based on the test's ability to detect drug use. The drug-detection window (DDW) for urine tests is one to three days. Therefore, testing every three or four days will detect most drug use. If such a test were part of a random drug-testing program, with the frequency of testing each individual averaging twice a month, then urine tests would be an effective way to gather drug-use information while discouraging use, since offenders would never know when they might be called to come in and provide a urine sample.

The DDW for oral fluids is twelve to twenty-four hours. These tests will need to be administered daily to detect the majority of drug use. Sweat patches detect drug use over two weeks, but they do so prospectively. Hair has the longest DDW, with typical analyses covering the last ninety days of drug use, minus the week just before the hair is cut.

These DDWs can then be used to calculate how often a particular type of test must be administered in order to have complete coverage and detect any drug use over a specified length of time. If, for example, a drug court was interested in monitoring drug use over a thirty-day period, a total of ten urine tests, two sweat-patch tests, thirty oral-fluids tests, or one hair test would have to be conducted to cover every day during that period.

As mentioned earlier, randomized testing can reduce the frequency of testing and overall cost without hindering overall effectiveness. The unpredictability of randomized testing is an incentive for abstinence because offenders have no idea when they will be tested next. When offenders begin monitoring, they are at a high probability of relapsing and beginning drug use again. However, after an extended period of monitoring—for instance, after two years on probation and at least twelve months of negative drug tests—that offender might be placed on a less frequent monitoring schedule. Therefore, random testing on an average of four times a month at the beginning of monitoring would be one way to cover most of the time, detect most drug use, and still motivate people to stay clean since the time of the next drug test cannot be predicted. After two years of monitoring and twelve months of drug-free urine samples have been obtained, monitoring could be reduced to one or two random urine tests per month and still achieve high compliance while reducing overall drug-testing program costs.

> Randomized testing can reduce the frequency of testing and overall cost without hindering overall effectiveness.

Marijuana (and its psychoactive component THC) presents a special challenge since, even after weeks of abstinence after heavy, long-term use, the urine may still test positive. Because THC is stored in the body's fat cells, it can take several weeks for the body to get rid of it. And for certain obese people, it can take even longer. Therefore, when offenders under community release are first tested, they are likely to test positive for marijuana even though they may not have used for several weeks. It would be possible to see what would normally be a gradual decline in the levels of THC in their urine; however, this type of test is rarely done because of its expense. Courts will generally ignore all such positive results for marijuana for at least the first month.

Random drug-testing programs can lower costs while preserving the deterrence of a more frequent testing program, but two important factors must be taken into account: frequency and true randomness. If the random program is designed so that only one sample is taken on average each month, then once that sample has been collected, offenders may be tempted to begin using drugs, guessing that it will probably be a long time before they are tested again. Therefore, to be effective, the random-testing program must be frequent enough that getting urine tested on any given day of any given week is a perceived possibility. The program must also be truly random in that even if an offender is tested on a Monday, he or she might just as easily be tested on the next day, Tuesday, as on any other day of the week. The moment an offender can guess when he or she will be tested is the moment the random-testing program's usefulness is dramatically diminished.

> The moment an offender can guess when he or she will be tested is the moment the random-testing program's usefulness is dramatically diminished.

Random-Testing Options

Several options exist for employing random testing. A correctional facility can choose not to employ random testing, can create or purchase software to manage random testing, or can contract with an outside agency to conduct random testing.

Nonrandom Testing

The most common method for setting the frequency of nonrandom testing is by correctional staff's choice. Many problems arise with nonrandom testing that becomes routine and is not driven by suspicion or evidence of possible drug use in a particular offender. For example, when a probation officer predictably tests all his parolees on Wednesday, it is easy for offenders to beat the drug test by not using drugs two to three days prior to the test. To maintain consistency and effectiveness, it is best to employ a truly random tracking system.

Random-Testing Software

Program directors or DTCs can develop their own in-house system using a software program to track drug testing or purchase an existing software program. The system must be able to track the following:

- who is being tested
- the duration of the test
- the random frequency of testing
- which offender belongs to which probation officer

The program should also be able to do the following:

- print test results and reports on suspicious use or failure to test
- produce annual reports and summaries
- print labels for bottles for multiple drug tests

Finally, the computer program should be user friendly. Having a system that is cumbersome and difficult to administer is counter-productive.

Good software is well worth the investment. It has the capacity to track all of this information with ease and accuracy. Software is constantly being developed. We suggest that you check for new software to manage drug testing; major laboratories and test-kit manufacturers are good places to start.

Contracting with an Outside Agency

Several outside agencies provide random drug testing. Many testing companies set up random testing at their own test sites throughout the nation. For urine tests, many testing companies use sites that are SAMHSA certified, employing certified collectors and following standard chain-of-custody procedures in sample collection. These companies can provide the necessary information and test results within twenty-four hours, allowing correctional facilities to track parolees and other community corrections offenders and monitor compliance through immediate updates on a Web site or via modem access.

> Contracting with an outside agency is advised when tracking the information and managing offenders overwhelms staff.

Contracting with an outside agency is advised when tracking the information and managing offenders overwhelms staff. Results are delivered in a timely fashion—soon enough to intervene with a relapsing offender. The cost is usually more than on-site testing and management, but if the funds can be allocated to this effort, it is worth it and certainly better than not having drug testing at all. A consideration is whether the test sites are accessible to offenders who may have transportation issues. This is a common excuse for not giving a drug-test sample on schedule, and it can be a valid justification or manipulation to avoid detection. In-house testing by an outside agency reduces the number of excuses and minimizes confrontations.

How to Buy Drug Tests

Buying drug tests is a little like buying a car or a ticket for an airplane. There is no one price, and there is no one right deal. The best answer to the question "What does it cost?" is "It depends." Our recommendation is that each correctional facility use all four major matrices for drug testing: urine, hair, oral fluids, and sweat patches. Each facility will want to have access to on-site test kits for urine and oral-fluids testing and laboratory-based testing for all four matrices. The facility will need to have procedures for confirming any screening test that is positive, even though the confirming tests for all four matrices will be used infrequently. It is desirable to retain positive samples when the offender disputes the result so that a retest can be done later.

> Buying drug tests is a little like buying a car or a ticket for an airplane. There is no one price, and there is no one right deal. The best answer to the question "What does it cost?" is "It depends."

Lack of resources to purchase adequate drug testing is a frequent complaint and a serious dilemma for many correctional facilities. It requires some ingenuity to get around the overwhelming obstacles related to cost, but there are ways to do it without jeopardizing the quality of the drug-testing program. This is what we mean when we recommend smarter drug testing. Most companies that sell drug tests are flexible with pricing. Quantity or volume reduces the cost per drug test. The more tests the facility orders, the lower the rate. A typical five-panel urine test with confirmation costs about $10 per panel. When a facility orders a large volume, the price may be reduced. This is true with all forms of drug testing. To reduce cost per test, the program director or DTC can consider collaborating with other agencies to increase the volume of the order. The DTC can collaborate with organizations that do their own drug testing, such as other probation departments, social-service agencies, other parole agencies, treatment facilities, or county or state mental-health agencies. He or she may negotiate a contract rate with a drug-testing company for a lower rate on laboratory-based toxicology services or to purchase a large volume of drug-test kits. If several agencies purchase drug-test kits together, the volume discount may require that the drug tests be delivered to one site and then distributed to each agency according to need.

Every correctional facility should have access to both on-site and laboratory-based testing, and every correctional facility should use urine, hair, oral-fluids, and sweat-patch tests. No one drug test is better than the others in all applications, and having access to all of them will greatly enhance the program's success. Diversity of testing may, however, operate against the desire of the program to get volume discounts. It may be that the volume discounts are only available for those tests used most often, and the program must pay full retail price for the other tests. Regardless, we recommend that the program use them to enhance the overall effectiveness of their drug-testing operations. In many correctional facilities, the most commonly used tests are on-site urine tests with a panel of five or six drugs. The second most common test is often an on-site oral-fluids test. Hair tests and laboratory-based testing for confirmation and for a broader range of drugs than is available with typical on-site tests come next in many correctional settings.

There are hundreds of potential suppliers of urine tests, a few providers of hair and oral-fluids tests, and, as of the writing of this manual, only one supplier for sweat-patch tests. The only tests approved for federal workplace tests are the urine laboratories listed on the SAMHSA Web site. These laboratories are subject to rigorous

> Every correctional facility should have access to both on-site and laboratory-based testing, and every correctional facility should use urine, hair, oral-fluids, and sweat-patch tests.

federal review, so they are a good place to start when thinking about laboratory-based urine-test providers.

Providers of on-site urine tests and other tests should be approved by the Food and Drug Administration. Check with your state and local drug-abuse offices to get information about approved laboratories and approved drug-test kits. Local suppliers of urine testing often have an advantage over national suppliers in terms of customer service. Remember, the program is buying more than just the test cups; it is buying the services, the support, and ultimately the skill in doing the analysis. We recommend that program staff become familiar with several providers and listen to what they have to say about their products and about competing products. Talk to other correctional facilities in your area. Listen to what they have to say about the providers of their drug testing. Get in touch with major employers in your area to see whom they use and what their experiences have been. When you go to local or national corrections conferences, network with some of the leading correctional facilities in your area or nationally to hear how they handle drug testing. Ask them about pricing and how they have made their deals.

> Providers of on-site urine tests and other tests should be approved by the Food and Drug Administration.

When considering a new provider of tests, request a side-by-side test of the new product with the one you are now using. Since you will have few positive tests of people who have been monitored for a long time, do the side-by-side comparison with your intake tests, which are far more likely to be positive. The biggest problem with tests is not that they give false-positive results, meaning that they identify drugs when no drugs are in the sample. This does not occur often, but when it does, it is easily identified through confirmatory testing. A false-negative result, meaning the test fails to identify drugs in the sample when they are actually there at or above the standard cutoff levels, is far more difficult to identify. This all-too-common problem with tests can, however, be easily identified in the side-by-side comparison using your current test against the new product at intake and on other likely positive samples. When there's a discrepancy between the two tests, send the positive sample off for confirmation. If it confirms positive, the other test produced a false-negative result, which disqualifies that product. Your program needs to be able to accurately identify drug use with the drug tests. Products that cannot do that are no bargain, no matter how cheap they are.

You will also need to be able to identify a far wider range of drugs than the SAMHSA-5 on at least some of your drug tests. Only urine offers the widest range of drugs on its panel, although in the near future, the other matrices will do that as their markets enlarge. The DTC needs to establish procedures for instances when corrections staff and others should request testing for a broader range of drugs, including specific drugs known to be abused by individual offenders. This testing can be negotiated with your laboratory. Some new on-site test kits can test for a wider range of drugs, and those are a good option as well. But for the tough cases, you will need a laboratory that can help you on a special-order basis.

We recommend that purchasing decisions be reviewed annually because the drug-testing market is large and rapidly changing. The best deal and the best test today may be obsolete within a year or two. This will take some time, presumably by the DTC, but the cost savings for the correctional facility earned from being a wise consumer can be enormous. But also remember that even paying high prices for the testing options that you use infrequently is a bargain, because having those unique tests available, even if they are seldom used, will greatly enhance the effectiveness of your overall drug-testing operation.

> We recommend that purchasing decisions be reviewed annually because the drug-testing market is large and rapidly changing.

The correctional facility's drug-test-kit providers and the laboratories the facility uses are valuable allies in drug testing. Get to know their customer-support people. Call them with any questions you have. They have a high level of expertise. They are motivated to help their customers. Good providers of drug testing provide good customer support. Use that support wisely and often. It is usually better to have the DTC contact these people, however, rather than individual staff members, because the DTC can often answer a staff member's questions without turning to customer support.

How Aggressive Should a Drug-Screening Program Be?

It's best to be as aggressive as possible in the implementation of a drug-testing program. We also recommend that drug tests be used at all stages of the criminal justice process: with volunteer arrestees and detainees at the pretrial stage; with court-ordered offenders at the conviction and incarceration stage; and with court-supervised community-released offenders, including probation, parole, and drug courts. The urgency of the drug problem in this country's criminal justice population, where more than half are using an illegal drug, demands the full use of this potent resource. The urgency of this situation demands an aggressive implementation of a drug-testing protocol.

> It's best to be as aggressive as possible in the implementation of a drug-testing program.

What to Do with a Positive Drug Test

For offenders, the results of a positive drug test are typically reported to the court. However, professionals working as probation and parole officers have discretion in how to handle a positive test result. As the earlier example of Tom demonstrated (see chapter 3), the probation officer understood that Tom had been working the system by abstaining from drug use just before his scheduled appointments and urine tests. As a result, Tom had what appeared to be an excellent record of negative test results. When another test was used, in that case a hair test, Tom's results came back positive. The probation officer did not immediately arrest Tom on a probation violation, but rather indicated that from then on a new test would be used and that Tom would no longer be able to hide his drug use. This advance warning of how the results of a more sensitive test will be used isn't just a compassionate response. It also recognizes that Tom has the capacity to limit his use over the short term to avoid detection and will now be encouraged to do the same over a longer term. In this way, the probation officer can continue to keep Tom out of an overcrowded jail and in the community, where he can provide for his family.

6

■　■　■　■　■

Problem Solving for Drug Tests
in Correctional Settings

While drug testing can sound simple, the interpretation of a drug-test result can be both confusing and inaccurate. Some problems come up repeatedly, while other problems are far less common. In this chapter, we address some of those common problems.

We begin by restating two fundamental facts about drug testing. First, drug tests identify the recent use of the specific drug or drugs included in the test panel. They do not identify impairment, addiction, or any of the many physical and psychological effects of drug use. They do not identify recent use of drugs that were not included in the test panel. Drug tests do not identify low levels of use or drug use in the remote past. Second, a negative drug test does not mean that the tested person did not recently use alcohol or other drugs. In other words, a positive drug test, correctly interpreted, means that recent use of the identified drug has occurred in the tested subject, nothing more and nothing less. A negative drug test only shows that the drugs that were tested for on the panel used in the particular drug test were not detected at or above the cutoff levels used in that test. A negative drug test cannot prove that a substance was never ingested.

Cheating

The most common and yet most serious problem with drug tests today is cheating. Cheating is defined as any of a large number of strategies drug users use to produce a negative drug test even when they have recently used drugs that are potentially identified by the drug-test panel. Drug users, especially drug users in the criminal justice system, have great incentives to cheat on drug tests.

Cheating has been a problem since the beginning of widespread drug testing four decades ago. In those days, the only drug tests that were commonly run were urine tests, and these tests were mostly very insensitive thin-layer chromatography. Since that time, tests have grown more sensitive, and the technology has evolved to the current standard of the immunoassay screen, followed (for samples that test positive) by the confirming GC/MS tests. Cheating on drug tests was common four decades ago. It is even more common today despite the large improvement in drug-testing technology. It is the desire to avoid consequences that keeps cheating a constant.

The two most simple and effective ways to cheat on urine drug tests are to submit someone else's urine as your own or to dilute your urine with water or some other liquid to bring the level of the drug in the urine below the cutoff used on the drug test. Dilution of the urine sample can occur in two ways: the tested person can add water to his or her urine sample, or more subtly and more difficult to detect, the tested person can drink a lot of fluid in the hour before the test so that the urine itself is diluted.

To reduce cheating, the standard procedure since the beginning of testing has been to have a staff member of the testing program directly observe the urine coming out of the tested person and into the collection cup. This unpleasant and socially stigmatized job is built into routine drug testing to ensure that the sample comes from the tested person and that nothing but urine has been put into the collection cup. This approach does not reduce cheating by consuming large volumes of water just before the test. To overcome that cheating strategy, it is necessary to have a staff person accompany the tested person from the time that person knows a drug test is coming until the sample is collected.

> The two most simple and effective ways to cheat on urine drug tests are to submit someone else's urine as your own or to dilute your urine with water or some other liquid.

When drug testing came out of drug-treatment programs and into the workplace in the 1980s, direct observation was considered a privacy violation. But where direct observation is not used, cheating is an even bigger problem. The criminal justice system has always directly observed the collection of urine samples, which is a big advantage in terms of reducing cheating.

Since all drug testing begins with the collection of the specimen, an important practical aspect of drug screening is the necessity of maintaining the chain of custody of the specimen, because the specimen is typically collected in one location but sent to a separate location for testing. The most important reason to perform direct observation of urine collections is to establish the chain of custody of that sample. Since the urine is potentially actual evidence in criminal court (at a probation hearing, for example), it is governed by the Federal Rules of Evidence. To be admissible, evidence must be relevant, material, and competent. Relevance and materiality of urine in a probation hearing is obvious to offer proof of compliance (or non-compliance) of a "no-use" condition of probation. But evidence must be real or authentic as well (Federal Rules of Evidence 901). A chain of custody establishes the whereabouts of the evidence at all times. Proper documentation following direct observation meets the burden of demonstrating that urine samples will be admissible in the courtroom. The chain of custody for a sample is the procedure that assures the court that the urine sample belongs to the person in question and that no one has added any substance to that evidence.

Almost as problematic as not observing collection of urine samples, even in the criminal justice system, has been the resistance of staff to do the dirty-seeming job of observing urine collection. Once the directly observed urine collection is given up or vigilance is not maintained, the possibilities for cheating expand exponentially.

When drug testing became more commonplace, an entire industry developed to "beat" the drug test. In 1986, political activist Abbie Hoffman wrote his now-classic book *Steal This Urine Test: Fighting Drug Hysteria in America* to encourage cheating on drug tests. He

> Since all drug testing begins with the collection of the specimen, an important practical aspect of drug screening is the necessity of maintaining the chain of custody of the specimen.

singled out the first author of this manual, *Drug Testing in Correctional Settings*, as one of the "gang of four" then bringing drug testing into the American workplace. Since that time, the Internet has taken over the role of marketing an ever-increasing number of sometimes highly sophisticated strategies for cheating drug tests. Take a look for yourself at the mind-boggling variety of offerings now available to cheat on drug tests.

Even direct observation of urine collections is no guarantee against cheating. A problem can occur when a single staff member is assigned the unpleasant job of observing urine collection. This person is subject to bribery by often-desperate clients. Even more common are the almost inevitable lapses in the vigilance of the staff member observing the urine collection since the precise visual connection to the process of urination is not easily maintained, especially when a large number of people are being screened in a short period of time, as is often the case in the criminal justice system. Another common problem occurs when agencies in the criminal justice system rely on drug-testing results administered in some other agency, including drug-treatment programs or the workplace. Many of these other sites do not observe collections at all, and when they do claim to observe collection, they do not do a good job of it. For this reason, it is desirable to have some or even all of the criminal justice drug testing done in the criminal justice programs themselves. That way, the test results are far more reliable.

A common way to discourage adulteration by dilution is to collect the samples in bathrooms that have the water turned off or that have blue dye put into the water in the toilet bowel so that adding water from that source is easily detected by visual inspection of the sample.

A common strategy for beating urine drug tests is for the tested person to come to the test with someone else's urine in a bag attached to plastic tubing that is run down to the usual place the urine leaves the tested person's body (i.e., the penis or vulva). By gently squeezing the bag, often strapped to the armpit or held between the buttocks, a stream of urine appears that is not easily distinguished

> Even direct observation of urine collections is no guarantee against cheating.

from naturally passed urine. Catching an offender who cheats in this way requires extra diligence on the part of the staff responsible for the collection.

Laboratories and the manufacturers of on-site urine test kits have worked to reduce cheating by employing a variety of strategies of varying effectiveness. One common strategy used today to reduce cheating on urine drug tests is to measure the temperature of the urine in the cup at the time of collection. If the temperature of the freshly provided urine sample is not close to the normal body temperature of 98.6° Fahrenheit, then the urine sample is declared to be an invalid specimen. When someone else's urine is brought in for purposes of cheating, it is often at room temperature. Room temperature is markedly lower than the average body temperature. When a urine sample is diluted with water, the temperature of the added water reduces the temperature of the submitted sample, making the cheating relatively easy to detect when the temperature of the sample is recorded.

In response to the use of techniques to measure the temperature of samples, would-be cheaters can buy tiny heaters and thermometers to ensure that the fake urine they provide is at precisely the right temperature before it is expelled into the collection cup. And, because carrying around human urine can be smelly and unpleasant, synthetic urine is now available. Synthetic urine is said to be identical to human urine and is not easily identified by laboratories or on-site test kits. What's more, synthetic urine has an indefinite shelf life—it does not spoil or give off odor when it is carried around for any length of time.

The simplest, easiest, and cheapest strategy to beat the urine drug test is still one of the best—drink a lot of water (a gallon or more) in the hour before giving the urine sample. In most drug-test samples, the level of drug is not far above the usual cutoff levels for the drug tests. In all of these cases, drinking a gallon or more of water, or any fluid containing water, before providing the urine sample successfully turns what would have been a positive drug-test result

> The simplest, easiest, and cheapest strategy to beat the urine drug test is still one of the best—drink a lot of water.

into a negative result by bringing the concentration down below the drug test's cutoff level.

Many of the techniques to beat drug tests sold on the Internet now involve consuming a lot of water, often mixed with one or more chemicals—euphemistically called "cleansing agents"—that are claimed to interfere with the testing process. These products designed to beat urine drug tests involve mixing the chemicals with lots of water because dilution is itself a good strategy to beat the urine drug tests. Of course, if the tested person has used a lot of drugs in the few hours just before the drug test, then dilution by drinking even a large quantity of water may not lower the level of the drug in the person's urine enough to produce a negative test.

Another common strategy for cheating on urine drug tests is to put a chemical into the urine test cup that confounds the initial immunoassay screening test. This strategy works even though the second, or confirming, drug test is unlikely to be fooled by the substance that is put into the urine, because if the screening test is negative, then no confirming test is done. Some chemicals frequently used to fool the screening tests are relatively easy for laboratories to identify, while newly emerging substances often succeed in thwarting the tests.

As urine drug tests have become more common so has the ingenuity of drug-test cheaters. There is money to be made in helping drug users beat drug tests in many settings, including the criminal justice system. This has resulted in an endlessly fascinating cat-and-mouse game. The drug users and the suppliers of products designed to thwart drug tests are trying to beat the tests while the testers and the suppliers of the drug tests are trying to protect the effectiveness of their tests. These two sides are continuously challenging each other's ingenuity and determination. As much as drug users are willing to pay for illegal drugs, they are willing to pay even more for reliable methods to beat drug tests.

For the urine drug-testing laboratories, detecting cheating has become a major new cost in the urine drug-test marketplace—a

> Another common strategy for cheating on urine drug tests is to put a chemical into the urine test cup that confounds the initial immunoassay screening test.

mature marketplace that is now largely driven by cost. This means that the laboratories are not eager to do the research needed to keep up with the well-funded deceivers. They are not even willing to do more than the cheapest and easiest tests to detect cheating. The drug-testing laboratories and the on-site drug-test manufacturers are not eager to add costs to their drug tests. Laboratories and on-site test manufacturers that add steps to detect cheating add to the costs of their tests. The drug-testing market punishes laboratories and test-kit manufacturers for innovations by almost always favoring the lowest cost provider. This market calculation would change if the federal government mandated effective strategies to identify and thwart cheating on urine drug testing, but the government has been unwilling to do this.

The manufacturers and the laboratories have limited incentives to detect cheating since the buyers of drug tests, agencies in the criminal justice system, have no way to know whether the urine drug tests they buy are resistant to cheating or not. The problem of perverse financial incentives is made worse by the fact that everyone in the drug-testing field has built-in, financially driven incentives to want more negative and fewer positive drug-test results. Surely drug users want more negative tests, that much is obvious. What is not so obvious are the incentives favoring negative tests, even negative tests as the result of cheating, within the criminal justice system and in other programs using the drug tests and in the laboratories and drug-test-kit manufacturers.

The criminal justice agencies want negative drug-test results. More negative tests mean fewer offenders needing more intensive services. For the laboratories doing the drug tests, the lower the level of positive drug-test results, the fewer tests that have to be confirmed (the most expensive part of the usual drug-test system) and the fewer results that need to be submitted for medical review—also an expensive process. Since the rate of positive tests is also a measure of program performance in the criminal justice system, akin to academic achievement scores on standardized tests in schools, the more

> The criminal justice agencies want negative drug-test results. More negative tests mean fewer offenders needing more intensive services.

negative and the fewer positive urine drug tests programs have, the better the programs appear.

The market for products that promote cheating is highly fragmented, meaning many small suppliers make up the market. There is no equivalent of Microsoft or McDonald's in the drug-test-cheating market. Were this market concentrated in a few suppliers with a few mass-market products, it would be much easier for the laboratories to identify the specific strategies being used to cheat on drug tests. Today's market of products to cheat on urine drug tests is not only fragmented, but it is also constantly changing. Today's cheating strategies are likely to be gone in a year or two. These market factors—the large number of small suppliers of rapidly changing products—create major problems not only for criminal justice programs, but for drug abusers seeking to cheat on urine drug tests as well. Both the cheaters and the cheated have a hard time figuring out which cheating products work and which do not (many do not work). For this reason, whatever products drug users choose in attempting to beat a urine drug test are subject to a high degree of uncertainty. Since many drug users pass urine drug tests anyway, simply getting past a particular drug test on one occasion, despite recent drug use, is no guarantee that the same product will get those drug users successfully past the next drug test they take.

The most common techniques for cheating are all made more difficult—but never impossible—by vigilant supervision of the collection under direct observation. And an offender who isn't aware of an upcoming test cannot consume a large quantity of water in anticipation of that test. To effectively reduce the risk of cheating on urine drug tests, it is important that the tester not be subject to bribery and carefully and directly observe the urine going into the collection cups. The tester must carefully monitor to ensure that the donor does not put anything else in the cup other than his or her urine. It cannot be stressed enough that donors not know of an upcoming test until they are under supervision so they do not have time to purchase a fake urine sample, equipment to cheat, or material to slip into the

> The most common techniques for cheating are all made more difficult—but never impossible—by vigilant supervision of the collection under direct observation.

collection cup with the urine, or have time to drink a large amount of fluid.

In court-ordered drug treatment, when the clients come to their clinics frequently or when they are in residential care, it is not difficult to meet all these requirements. Under those circumstances, drug tests can be administered on an unannounced and random basis. Even then, however, vigilance is needed, including careful implementation of the drug testing so that the tested person is not inadvertently allowed to get material for cheating or consume lots of fluid before the test. In the criminal justice system, where contact is less frequent, it is not possible to meet these conditions. Offenders then have ample warning of when they may be tested, permitting lots of time to prepare to cheat. They also have another way to beat the test; this involves refraining from drug use for a few days prior to scheduled visits that include urine collection. This is a successful cheating strategy because most drugs have a drug-detection window of one to three days. While some of the physiologically addicted offenders, heroin addicts for example, will not be able to abstain from use for three days without being very sick, many other drug users can easily time their drug use to avoid detection. There are two good ways to solve this problem. The first is a random drug test at an unexpected time. You could call the parolee or probationer and require him or her to come in within a few hours for a drug test. However, this still permits the person to consume an adulterant or to drink excessive amounts of fluid. An unannounced visit to the offender that includes a drug test will solve this problem. The second way to overcome the problem of the regularly scheduled visit at which tests are taken is to conduct a hair test, analyzing the half-inch of hair closest to the head; this covers a month of possible drug use. Hair testing will not identify marijuana use at a frequency of less than two to three times a week, but it will identify other drug use in the prior month at a lower frequency. Hair testing is not subject to cheating by excessive water consumption or by other strategies that work for urine tests. Longer time periods, of course, can be studied

> The second way to overcome the problem of the regularly scheduled visit at which tests are taken is to conduct a hair test, analyzing the half-inch of hair closest to the head; this covers a month of possible drug use.

with longer hair samples; as hair grows half an inch a month, a one-and-one-half-inch hair sample covers the prior ninety days.

With respect to the problem of bribery, it is desirable to have more than one person on the staff of the testing program doing the observation and to randomly and unpredictably rotate the staff doing the observation. This way, neither the staff nor the offenders can be sure of a particular pairing of an offender and an observer until the time of the test.

There are several strategies for detecting some types of cheating after it occurs on urine tests. One way to detect cheating is to have the testing laboratory conduct confirming GC/MS tests on some samples that are negative on the screening test. However, these confirming tests, which are much less subject to cheating, are expensive. In addition, large numbers of negative tests must be submitted to these confirming tests to detect cheating, since in most drug-testing programs the large majority of urine samples are truly negative. If only 5 percent of urine drug tests are initially found to be positive for recent drug use, and if half of the positives are turned negative by cheating, then twenty negative samples, on average, would have to be tested to find just one sample that had tested negative on the screen despite the presence of an identifiable drug at or above the standard cutoff level.

The most common way to cheat on a urine test is to consume a lot of liquids, and while it is easy for both on-site and laboratory testing to detect a diluted sample, it's not as easy to prove that this represents an attempt to cheat. The testing laboratory can "normalize" the urine from diluted to normal concentration by adjusting the test level for the level of creatinine in the urine. Very diluted urine (because of excessive hydration) has low creatinine levels. The laboratory can adjust the threshold level of a drug found below the cutoff, bringing it back to the level it would have been if the fluid had not been consumed. There is a proposal to normalize diluted urine sample results for federally sanctioned urine drug laboratories. This strategy is not now generally available. At this time, normalization of

> There are several strategies for detecting some types of cheating after it occurs on urine tests.

diluted specimens cannot be provided with on-site urine drug-testing kits. Laboratories can test for some of the more common chemicals used to fool the screening immunoassay tests, but these tests to identify chemicals used to cheat are expensive. Because so many different chemicals are used to cheat, the laboratories have to test for each potential cheating chemical separately, rendering this solution impractical.

There is another, much more powerful strategy available to reduce cheating on drug tests. This strategy is even more effective and a lot easier to manage than direct observation of urine collection and careful management of the tested person after that person knows he or she will be tested. The strategy is to use alternative samples—hair, oral fluids, and sweat—all virtually immune to cheating. This means that if a hair, oral-fluids, or sweat sample is taken instead of a urine sample, then all of the strategies used to cheat on a urine test that we have described—strategies that are now common—are completely ineffective. If the people being drug tested do not know whether they will be given a urine, hair, oral-fluids, or sweat test on any given drug-testing experience, it is a lot more difficult for them to prepare to cheat.

> There is another, much more powerful strategy available to reduce cheating on drug tests.

Using an unannounced mix of drug tests also overcomes the often problematic reliance on the staff person who has to vigilantly and directly observe the urine coming out of the donor and into the cup. Staff members much prefer to collect hair, oral fluids, or sweat than to directly observe urine collection. The collection of hair, oral fluids, and sweat does not take place in a bathroom or involve inspection of "private parts" of the body. With these alternative samples, it is not necessary for the laboratory to test for confounding substances. There is no need to measure the temperature of the sample. Consuming large quantities of water does not invalidate the test result for any sample except a urine sample.

The criminal justice system program that uses all the major testing methods on a basis that cannot be predicted by the offenders—on-site and laboratory-based testing, plus testing of urine as well as hair, oral fluids, and sweat—over time can easily compare the rates of positive results on the various testing methods to determine which is the most effective in detecting recent drug use. Even if one drug-test method is clearly superior to the others, we suggest that the program continue to use a mix of methods to discourage cheating. If the program does anything the same way over and over again in an entirely predictable fashion, the potential for cheating goes up since the opportunity for motivated, smart, and inventive drug users to cheat goes up in proportion to the predictability of a drug-testing strategy. To stay ahead, the agency has to keep one step ahead of the offenders.

> Even if one drug-test method is clearly superior to the others, we suggest that the program continue to use a mix of methods to discourage cheating.

Claims of Secondhand Drug Exposure

While far less common than in workplace drug testing, it is possible to face a claim that a positive drug test was the result of passive or innocent exposure, for example, from being around someone else who was smoking marijuana or cocaine or being slipped the drug in food or drink.

This entire manual could be devoted to the science behind the thousands of different scenarios that have come up in drug-testing programs. A favorite is a probationer who claimed his positive cocaine test resulted from the fact that his son cooked cocaine to make crack as part of his work as a drug dealer. To do his cooking, the man's son used the pan that the probationer used to prepare his oatmeal for breakfast.

> There is no scenario that would lead to a positive test on an innocent basis for any specimen and for any drug.

While tales like these abound, there is no scenario that would lead to a positive test on an innocent basis for any specimen and for any drug. There is one exception to this statement, and that is the legitimate medical prescription of controlled substances, which are identified on drug tests. Programs need to be able to follow up such claims and to deal with them appropriately.

In the criminal justice system, especially, there are two factors that make the innocent-exposure argument far less relevant than it is in drug-treatment, workplace, or school-based drug testing. In the criminal justice system, it is rare that a severe penalty will be given for a single positive drug test. More often, a series of positive tests will lead to serious consequences, making a single test result less important. In addition, for people in the criminal justice system, it is not "innocent" to be around people who are using illegal drugs.

However, if you come across a result that puzzles you, or if you are in serious doubt about the interpretation of a drug-test result, call your drug-testing laboratory or the manufacturer of the test kits you are using and ask for help. Most have toxicologists on staff who can help sort out the most difficult claims in scientific and convincing ways. If there is a dispute over a test result, record the thought process you used to come to the conclusion you reached so that the basis for your conclusion is documented. Do not be shy about getting more information if you have continuing doubts. Check with academic experts in toxicology at a local university or at a local police or medical laboratory. You can also call the American Society of Addiction Medicine (ASAM) to find a local medical review officer, a physician specially trained to interpret drug-test results. Contact information for ASAM is provided on page 106. In most settings, it is also easy enough to get another drug test if you need one. Drug abuse is almost never an isolated event. If the person is using a drug, that fact is likely to become evident with repeated drug testing.

> In most settings, it is also easy enough to get anther drug test if you need one.

The Poppy-Seed Problem

Heroin is made from morphine, which comes from the opium poppy. When the body breaks down heroin, the second metabolite is morphine. Drug tests usually identify morphine and not heroin since the heroin does not last long in the body and is in lower concentration in the urine. Drug tests, therefore, routinely identify morphine, the heroin metabolite, when the urine of heroin addicts is tested.

The poppy seeds in our foods have morphine in them in such low quantities that it has no biological effects, but it may be enough to give a positive urine drug test in the few hours after eating poppy seeds. Even the number of poppy seeds on a single bagel is enough to produce a positive urine drug test. This is not a "false positive," since the morphine is in the urine at or above the standard cutoff levels. In the workplace, where heroin use is less common than poppy-seed consumption and where the interpretation of test results is adjusted to prevent any mistaken attribution of drug abuse, the morphine-positive tests are virtually all reversed. This means that it is almost impossible for a heroin addict to be identified in routine workplace drug tests. In the criminal justice system, in contrast, where heroin use is far more common than poppy-seed use, a morphine positive is interpreted as a heroin positive. Offenders need to be warned about this fact so that they can avoid eating poppy seeds.

> There is not enough morphine in poppy-seed products to trigger positive results on oral-fluids, sweat, or hair tests.

In this instance, there is once again an advantage to using a sample other than urine. There is not enough morphine in poppy-seed products to trigger positive results on oral-fluids, sweat, or hair tests, plus all of these alternative specimens permit the identification of the first metabolite of heroin, 6-MAM, which is seldom found in urine samples. This specific metabolite is only present after heroin use, never after poppy-seed consumption.

Claims That Current Positive Drug Tests Are the Result of Long-Ago Drug Use

Urine tests detect drug use that occurred in the one to three days prior to the sample collection. There are a few exceptions to this, and they only apply to heavy drug users. For marijuana, a heavy user may stay positive at routine cutoff levels for up to two weeks or longer, although most heavy users are negative sooner than two weeks after they stop smoking marijuana. Some crack users also have very high levels of cocaine, and its major metabolites remain in their urine for a week or two after they stop using crack.

If, during repeated testing, there has been a negative test between two positive tests and/or if more than a couple of weeks have passed since the last admitted use, it is highly likely that there has been new use of the drug since the negative sample was provided. There are some rare exceptions to this rule, but it is a good place to start. If there is a reason to investigate a particular case further, we suggest you contact a toxicologist familiar with interpreting drug tests to sort out the facts of the case.

7

■ ■ ■ ■ ■

Evaluation, Research, and Additional Resources

In this chapter, we make suggestions on how evaluation can be done systematically in a way that benefits the offenders and the correctional program itself. A growing trend in the criminal justice system requires agencies to show the effectiveness of their law-enforcement programs by reporting outcome data. State and federal programs are being asked not only to verify effectiveness but also to have evidence-based approaches to law enforcement that have been shown to be effective through extensive research.

For example, the federally funded Weed and Seed demonstration program mandated that funded jurisdictions demonstrate how their strategies weeded out the drug sellers yet helped drug users get treatment and lowered drug use in the target communities. An effective drug-testing program that operated at the local jail and tracked results by zip code would contribute to this evaluation by demonstrating how use went down in that community while arrests for possession were going up. Policy assessment can also benefit public relations by demonstrating the effectiveness of a particular community-based operation that has been designed, for example, to eliminate drug sales in certain neighborhoods.

Not providing outcome data will often jeopardize the receipt of continued federal or state funding designated to run a specific community-based or even prison-based drug-elimination program. Collecting outcome data, on the other hand, could enhance the programs' competitive position in acquiring new grant monies to run such programs. For example, drug-court programs require weekly reports on how well clients are doing in treatment. A management information system could be used to track drug tests and treatment results, which are then summarized in an annual evaluation report. This information could be used as part of a national database to continue to justify the need for drug courts. Without this information, federal funding would cease to exist.

Setting up a protocol for drug testing for outcome data is fairly simple. What is required is a management information system that is practical, easy, and efficient. The agency needs a database program to track demographic information and drug-test results. Information to track includes date of entering the system, drug-test results, and criminal charges. Demographics such as age, gender, race, and zip code can also be tracked. A note of caution: since this policy assessment and testing program will rely on volunteers, individual identifiers should never be included in this research database. To do so would violate the arrestees' rights under the federal Health Insurance Portability and Accountability Act (HIPAA).

Correctional programs are usually underfunded. Every penny available to the program is plowed into the delivery of much-needed services. Evaluation and research are often put on the back burner given the tight budgets. Despite these budgets, it is shortsighted even for the most resource-poor correctional program not to do evaluation and research. In many communities, it is possible for the staff members responsible for evaluation and research—even if this is a part-time role—to leverage their efforts by involving students and faculty from local universities or other organizations interested in studying drug abuse in a correctional setting. It is also possible to get research funding from local nonprofit organizations to support research activities.

A staff member in the correctional system should be designated the research coordinator (RC). Although this is usually a part-time role in addition to other responsibilities, the RC's duties should include writing an annual report to the head of the correctional program or

> Setting up a protocol for drug testing for outcome data is fairly simple. What is required is a management information system that is practical, easy, and efficient.

to the agency responsible for the correctional program, describing in detail the evaluation and research activities that took place in the previous year and what is planned for the upcoming year. This report should include the following components:

- **Monthly drug-testing data for the previous year.** List the total number of drug tests given and the percentage that were negative and positive, making separate listings for random and for-cause drug tests. These positive tests can be broken down further to show how many drugs and what types of different drugs were detected. Monthly and annual drug-test results can be analyzed for each kind of test, reporting separately for urine, hair, oral-fluids, and sweat samples. Over the course of a single year, trend lines can be drawn with the monthly data. This basic report will give the program valuable data on which drugs are used, how often, and by whom.

- **A monthly tabulation of intake drug-test results.** These results should reflect the patterns of drug use in the community. They can be reported to the community and to agencies with special interest in this data, including health and law-enforcement agencies. This provides a way for a program to identify new drug-abuse trends in the community. This information can be used for an op-ed article in the local newspaper or reported to local health and law-enforcement officials.

Setting up a protocol for drug testing to achieve outcome data does not need to be complicated. Start by identifying one staff member as the designated RC. This could be the drug-testing coordinator (DTC). This person can be in charge of outcome data. First, you will need a management information system that is practical, easy, and efficient and includes a database program such as Microsoft Access to track information and drug-test results. Information that should be tracked includes the following:

- who is being tested
- the duration of the test
- the random frequency of testing
- which offender belongs to which probation officer

Setting up a protocol for drug testing to achieve outcome data does not need to be complicated.

The program should also be able to do the following:

- print test results and reports on suspicious use or failure to test
- produce annual reports and summaries
- print labels for bottles for multiple drug tests

Initial information should be gathered at the time of arrest. At this time, drug history, including the most recent level of use for the past thirty days, should be recorded. This includes use of alcohol and all forms of other drugs. A drug test should be administered sometime during the first week or at the initial intake session. This will establish a baseline. A regular testing protocol including a set frequency of sample collection should be established. That way, all offenders will receive the same protocol to keep the integrity of the data intact. Having one offender tested twice a month and another tested randomly once per week makes it impossible to compare the data. You can't compare apples to oranges in research.

If it is impossible to keep the frequency of collection consistent for offenders who are at low risk for drug use, hair analysis can be used. It would give you the information equal to weekly urine tests even if these offenders were only tested once every ninety days. Having a standard drug-testing protocol will make it easier to interpret your data and evaluate your program.

Once a baseline is established and offenders are being tested consistently, a follow-up drug test can be conducted, preferably six months after court-ordered treatment, by requiring the offender to come in for a drug test and interview. This information is critical in determining how well the person is doing after he or she has left the court-ordered treatment program. It helps to answer the question of whether the treatment episode was sufficient to sustain the person's recovery without further support.

The ideal for collecting outcome data is to see the offender individually. That way, you can observe his or her affect and physical appearance in conjunction to what is said. You can better evaluate

> Once a baseline is established and offenders are being tested consistently, a follow-up drug test can be conducted, preferably six months after court-ordered treatment.

the congruency between observable behaviors and what the person is reporting. You will also be able to collect a drug test to validate sobriety. Hair analysis will give you the most accurate information over the longest period of time: ninety days as opposed to one to three days for a urine sample. In addition to the drug tests, you may also want to use the Addiction Severity Index (ASI). This survey instrument is a good treatment evaluation tool to measure areas of improvement throughout a person's recovery. Abstinence is one way to measure success, but improvements in employment, education, health, psychosocial behavior, legal issues, and so on are even more impressive for those who are serving out their sentence in a community setting. The ASI will provide this information during this follow-up interview.

To have good outcome data, you do not have to evaluate everyone who goes through your correctional program. Randomizing 25 percent of your offenders for posttreatment evaluation will offer a good sample for assessing how well your program is performing and will reduce the cost of a follow-up survey.

> To have good outcome data, you do not have to evaluate everyone who goes through your correctional program.

Program evaluation can also compare previous services with new services. This may involve partial aspects of a program or an entire program. Drug testing can be used as a primary measurement of court-ordered treatment success. As you make changes and improvements in your correctional program throughout the year, drug-test results either validate or invalidate these changes.

Drug-testing costs need to be tracked. This should include direct costs of the drug tests themselves, as well as staff time devoted to the drug-testing process. Innovative solutions can be studied to keep these costs down. Random drug testing and use of hair testing instead of frequent urine tests for low-risk offenders allow the correctional program to stretch out the testing over longer periods of time, saving money over more frequent standard testing. The DTC should manage the random drug-testing schedule informing correctional staff when particular offenders need to be tested.

Support, Advice, and Additional Resources

The DTC should be the single point of contact within the program staff for issues related to drug testing. This is a big step toward keeping up with the rapidly evolving field of drug-testing technology and its many highly valuable applications in correctional settings.

The DTC should coordinate outreach efforts to other correctional and court-ordered drug-treatment programs. Scheduling quarterly meetings is a good way to provide collaboration opportunities and support to all staff members who are involved in the drug-testing process. Having speakers from both outside and inside the organization keeps interest up and brings in new information. By bringing in outside speakers, a drug-testing network can be established to include other community organizations. This is a great way to develop cooperative arrangements with other programs that will allow buying better services and products at lower costs.

> The DTC should be the single point of contact within the program staff for issues related to drug testing.

Experts at local universities who have an interest in drug testing in correctional settings can also be useful to the program by answering questions that arise. The medical review officers (MROs) in your community can be consulted regarding questionable drug-testing results. MROs can be found by contacting the American Society of Addiction Medicine (ASAM) at www.asam.org or (301) 656-3920. Whether the correctional program uses an MRO or not, it is useful to have an MRO that the DTC can call to discuss difficult or confusing drug-test results.

■   ■   ■

Some additional resources that can be helpful to the DTC include the following:

Center for Substance Abuse Treatment (CSAT)
http://csat.samhsa.gov

Drug and Alcohol Testing Industry Association (DATIA)
www.datia.org

Institute for a Drug-Free Workplace
www.drugfreeworkplace.org

Institute for Behavior and Health, Inc. (IBH)
www.ibhinc.org

National Association of State Alcohol and Drug Abuse Directors, Inc. (NASADAD)
www.nasadad.org

National Center on Addiction and Substance Abuse at Columbia University (CASA)
www.casacolumbia.org

National Clearinghouse for Alcohol and Drug Information (NCADI)
www.health.org

National Institute on Chemical Dependency (NICD)
www.ni-cor.com

Office of National Drug Control Policy (ONDCP)
www.whitehousedrugpolicy.gov

Substance Abuse and Mental Health Services Administration (SAMHSA)
www.samhsa.gov

Substance Treatment
www.substancetreatment.com

8

Conclusion

The criminal justice system is the last best hope for many addicted people to get well and to stay well. Prison is not the deepest "bottom" for addicted offenders—death is that bottom. Prison is, however, a very deep bottom for many people. For the criminal justice system to fulfill its twin roles of correction of offenders and protection of the community, the criminal justice system must maintain a drug-free standard that is enforced by frequent drug testing.

To be cost effective and mindful of seemingly perpetually strained budgets, this drug testing must be smart. That means using random testing calibrated to the risk of illegal drug use for each individual offender, and it means using the full range of modern drug tests, not only urine tests, but also testing of hair, oral fluids, and sweat. Beyond that, smart drug testing means careful choice of the drugs to be tested so the offender does not know which drugs will be identified with any particular drug test, and so that the range of drugs tested for is extensive. While it is true that just five drugs will capture most drug use of offenders (alcohol, marijuana, cocaine, heroin, and methamphetamine), it is also true that many other drugs are also used. The ability to detect the use of a wide range of abused drugs, not just the five most commonly used drugs, is vital to having the most cost-effective drug-abuse (and crime) prevention as a result of drug testing in the criminal justice system.

We have described how to use random testing and how to use drug tests other than urine tests. Some readers may conclude that we are anti–urine testing or that we are pro–hair or pro–oral-fluids testing. That conclusion is wrong. We are pro–drug testing. We want agencies of the entire criminal justice system to use the full range of drug-testing options that are now available. We recognize that urine tests are the most commonly used drug tests because they are more familiar and they are generally the least expensive on a per-test basis. We also recognize that it is easier to customize the drugs being tested for when looking for less commonly used drugs with urine tests than with alternative drug tests. We know on-site tests are especially valuable in the criminal justice system and that on-site drug-test options are available for urine and oral fluids but not for hair and sweat. We want everyone working in the criminal justice system to know more about the full range of drug-testing options and to be able to pick the one drug test that best fits each situation. Because most professionals in the criminal justice system are familiar with urine testing, and many people are not familiar with hair, oral-fluids, and sweat testing, we have emphasized these alternative drug tests.

> Some readers may conclude that we are anti–urine testing or that we are pro–hair or pro–oral-fluids testing. That conclusion is wrong. We are pro–drug testing.

We encourage each criminal justice system program to do evaluations of their drug-testing activities and to report these results to the public and to funding sources because we know from experience that these reports, based on the objective evidence produced by regular drug testing, will not only add to the knowledge about drug use in the community, but will also validate the work of the criminal justice system agency itself. Evaluation reports of drug-test results will also lead to improvements in the criminal justice system program and help identify more cost-effective ways to manage the agency's drug-testing program.

Our experience has shown us the ability of criminal justice system drug-testing programs to identify illegal drug use, to focus interventions when illegal drug use occurs, and to support and manage the essential programs of recovery. It is the experience of recovering from addiction, often sparked by the hard edge of the criminal justice system, that inspires us. We believe the experience of recovery in your offender population will inspire you in your work. For this goal of recovery to be achieved by more criminal offenders, it is essential that drug-testing programs in the criminal justice system work better and cheaper. We hope that you, after you have read this manual, are now better able to achieve this humanitarian goal in your program.

Our experience has shown us the ability of criminal justice system drug-testing programs to identify illegal drug use, to focus interventions when illegal drug use occurs, and to support and manage the essential programs of recovery.

Index

■   ■   ■

About the Authors

■ ■ ■

Robert L. DuPont, M.D.

Robert DuPont was the first director of the National Institute on Drug Abuse (NIDA) and the second White House Drug Czar. He began his career as director of Community Services for the District of Columbia Department of Corrections before founding the citywide Narcotics Treatment Administration (NTA). NTA was the inspiration for the federal government's massive commitment to addiction treatment in the early 1970s. He helped found the first universal drug-testing program for probation and pretrial release in the nation's capital in 1970.

DuPont was an early leader in the application of drug testing in many settings including drug-abuse treatment, the civilian workplace, and more recently in schools. He is also an extensively published author, with more than twenty professional books and monographs to his credit, including *The Selfish Brain: Learning from Addiction*, which was published in paperback by Hazelden.

DuPont has been a national leader in drug-abuse prevention and treatment for more than three decades, focusing on broadly based public health approaches to reducing illegal drug use. Since 1978, he has been president of the Institute for Behavior and Health, Inc. (www.ibhinc.org), a nonprofit organization devoted to drug-abuse policy. He is clinical professor of psychiatry at Georgetown University School of Medicine and vice president of Bensinger, DuPont, and Associates, a national organization devoted to workplace drug-abuse prevention, employee assistance programs, and the reduction of prescription drug abuse.

Thomas M. Mieczkowski, Ph.D.

Thomas Mieczkowski is a researcher and academic whose interests have included drug epidemiology and the validation of various drug-detection technologies. He has published numerous scholarly articles and book chapters. He has also published two books: *Drugs, Crime, and Social Policy: Research, Issues, and Concerns* and a book on bioassay technology entitled *Drug Testing Technology: Assessment of Field Applications*.

Since receiving his Ph.D. from Detroit's Wayne State University in 1985, Mieczkowski has received more than one million dollars in research funding. He is an active member of the International Association of Forensic Toxicologists, the British Academy of Forensic Sciences, the European Hair Research Society, and the American Society of Criminology. And he serves as editor of the *International Journal of Drug Testing*.

Mieczkowski is also an active consultant for both government and private agencies. He has consulted for the National Institute on Drug Abuse, the National Institute of Justice, the American Probation and Parole Association, the American Correctional Association, the American College of Occupational and Environmental Medicine, the Justice Research and Statistics Association, and several private corporations, including Michelin and Anheuser-Busch. He has lectured internationally, including invited lectures at the Royal Society of Medicine in London and the National Youth Center in Tokyo, and to a consortium of police executives in the United Arab Emirates.

Richard A. Newel, Ph.D.

Richard Newel has been conducting research in drug abuse and drug detection for nearly twenty-five years. He is an author on more than forty publications and professional papers devoted to drug testing in general and hair testing in particular. Currently at the University of South Florida, Newel has taught graduate-level counselor education classes in substance abuse as well as introductory classes in forensics in criminology. He has also recently been asked to provide testimony before the United States Congress on the Department of Health and Human Services' policy for Federal Workplace Drug-Testing Programs as well as in the Food and Drug Administration's hearings on testing for drugs of abuse.